Shared Care in Mental Health

by
Dr Laurence Mynors-Wallis MA, DM, MRCP, MRCPsych
Consultant Psychiatrist, Alderney Hospital, Dorset, UK

Dr Michael Moore BMedSci, BM BS, MRCP, FRCGP, DRCoG
General Practitioner, Three Swans Surgery, Salisbury, UK

Mr Jon Maguire RNMH, RMN, DipIMHW, MSc (Econ)
Community Health Nurse, Brasenose Centre, Oxford, UK

Mr Timothy Hollingbery BA, MSc, CPsychol, AFBPsS
Consultant Clinical Psychologist, St Ann's Hospital, Dorset, UK

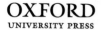

OXFORD
UNIVERSITY PRESS

Great Clarendon Street, Oxford OX2 6DP

Oxford University Press is a department of the University of Oxford.
It furthers the University's objective of excellence in research, scholarship,
and education by publishing worldwide in

Oxford New York

Auckland Bangkok Buenos Aires Cape Town Chennai
Dar es Salaam Delhi Hong Kong Istanbul Karachi Kolkata
Kuala Lumpur Madrid Melbourne Mexico City Mumbai Nairobi
São Paulo Shanghai Taipei Tokyo Toronto

Oxford is a registered trade mark of Oxford University Press
in the UK and in certain other countries

Published in the United States
by Oxford University Press Inc., New York

© Oxford University Press, 2002

The moral rights of the author have been asserted

Database right Oxford University Press (maker)

First published 2002

Reprinted 2003

British Library Cataloguing in Publication Data
Data available

Library of Congress Cataloging in Publication Data
Data available

ISBN 0 19 852545 1

10 9 8 7 6 5 4 3 2 1

Typeset by Top Draw Design
Printed in Great Britain
on acid-free paper by Biddles Ltd, www.biddles.co.uk

Contents

Introduction

Patients in primary care present with complex problems and not neat diagnostic labels. Moreover the problems are often overlapping, poorly defined and hard to categorize. The GP may not arrive at a clearly defined diagnosis but uses a series of evolving operational diagnoses which guide treatment and management decisions. We have used a problem-orientated approach rather than a cosy disease-orientated approach but have used diagnostic categories when it seemed helpful. GPs will be familiar with the patients in their consulting rooms who, although having psychosocial problems, do not have a 'treatable mental illness'. These patients nevertheless pose management problems and consume time and resources. We have tried to include some management strategies for these often difficult patients.

The term 'shared care' means different things on either side of the primary care, secondary care divide. Secondary care may have unrealistic expectations about what is possible in primary care, and are on occasion insensitive as to the knowledge that the primary care team bring to a case. Primary care may be prickly about what they see as an attempt to foist yet more work upon an already over-burdened service. We believe there should be a blurring of boundaries between primary and secondary care and for many patients there should be a team approach to care. Our view of shared care is that at different times, patients with mental health problems will have varying proportions of their care delivered within primary or secondary services. The advent of primary care trusts may alter the concept of shared care further with a move to service specification and pathways of care. However, even in well-integrated services it will be difficult to be overly precise as patients do not necessarily follow the agreed pathways of care.

We believe shared care means not only care shared between primary and secondary care but also utilizing the skills of the non-medical members of the primary health care team. It has been shown that nurses are able to deliver brief psychological treatments in primary care and should probably be used more widely in such a role. The majority of psychiatric morbidity is represented by chronic disorders which vary in severity and impact over time. These disorders cause a burden of symptoms for the individual and a burden of management for professionals. The number and variety of healthcare professionals involved will wax and wane as symptoms and coping skills worsen or improve with life events. Shared care means sharing the burden of care; essential to this is:

- Good communication.
- Clear lines of responsibility.
- Utilizing the knowledge and skills of other team members and recognizing when to involve them.
- Good working relationships which are worth more than any number of agreed policies and protocols.

The chapters are set out to address 'problems': each starts with a hit list of the information and strategies we are trying to provide. Each chapter follows a standard format:

- Epidemiology (including morbidity).
- Recognition and diagnosis.
- Management in primary care.
- When to refer.
- What to expect from secondary services.

Within management we have concentrated on what is feasible within primary care. We have attempted to provide clear advice and, in particular, detailed descriptions of psychological interventions that may be of value and which are possible within a normal consultation. We have provided illustrative vignettes both to highlight key points in practice and to provide discussion points for learning and teaching. Many chapters could provide a book in their own right and we have provided suggested reading if you find your appetite whetted. The book is designed to be dipped into when faced with a problem in practice and we hope that you find it a useful resource.

Abbreviations

AIDS   acquired immunodeficiency syndrome

AUDIT   Alcohol Use Disorders Identification Test

BNF   British National Formulary

bd   twice a day

CBT   cognitive behaviour therapy

CDT   carbohydrate deficient transferin

CEBM   Centre for Evidence Based Mental Health

CMHT   community mental health team

CPA   Care Programme Approach

DSH   deliberate self-harm

DSM-IV   Diagnostic and Statistical Manual of Mental Disorders

DVLA   Driver and Vehicle Licensing Agency

ECG   electrocardiogram

ECT   electroconvulsive therapy

GABA   gamma-aminobutyric acid

GGT   gamma-glutamyltransferase

GHQ   General Health Questionnaire

GP   general practitioner

5-HT   serotonin (5-hydroxytryptamine)

HIV   human immunodeficiency virus

ICD-10   International Classification of Disease – Version 10

IHD   ischaemic heart disease

MAOIs   monoamine oxidase reuptake inhibitors

MCV   mean corpuscular volume

MDMA   methylenedioxymethamphetamine (ecstasy)

MMSE   mini mental state examination

NA   noradrenaline

NSAIDS   non-steroidal anti-inflammatory drugs

OCD   obsessive compulsive disorder

PTSD   post-traumatic stress disorder

SSRIs   specific serotonin reuptake inhibitors

TCAs   tricyclic antidepressants

tds   three times a day

TFT   thyroid function tests

WHO   World Health Organization

chapter 1

The depressed patient

IN THIS CHAPTER

- Recognition and diagnosis of depression.
- Who and how to treat with antidepressants.
- When and how to discontinue antidepressants.
- Use of simple brief psychological interventions.
- Risk assessment and when to refer.

INTRODUCTION

The appropriate management of the depressed patient is probably the key psychiatric skill for the GP to master. Not only are depressive disorders very common (1 in 10 consulting patients), but also effective primary care-based treatments can make a marked impact on patient morbidity and recovery.

Depression is without question a disorder of primary care with approximately 90% of cases seen and treated without specialist referral. However, the GP has long been berated for not recognizing cases of depressive disorder, and then not adequately treating those cases which are recognized. This chapter sets out a pragmatic approach to diagnosis and treatment, which seeks to empower rather than criticize the GP. Guidance is given (evidence based where possible) to support the key management steps.

EPIDEMIOLOGY

There is an increasing prevalence of depression from community studies (2–4%) to primary care (5–10%) and secondary care (10–14%) (Katon and Schulberg, 1992). Given that depressive disorders are on a continuum, for every clear-cut 'case' there will be a further two patients with fewer or less severe symptoms.

Patients in primary care rarely have depressive symptoms alone: approximately 60% will have at least one other psychiatric disorder; depression is particularly associated with anxiety disorders and alcohol dependence. Depressive disorders also commonly accompany physical illnesses, especially cardiovascular disease, cancer and chronic pain.

Table 1.1. Epidemiology of depressive disorders

- Lifetime prevalence: approximately 20%
- Risk factors include:
  - being female (twice the rates for men)
  - family history
  - previous depression
  - chronic physical illness
  - stressful life events
  - alcohol or substance abuse
  - family disadvantages in early life
- Peak age of onset: 20–40 years
- Prevalence in primary care: 1 in 10 consulting patients (approximately half of whom will benefit from antidepressant medication)
- Suicide 20 x population average

Clinical course

Depression is often a chronic illness, although many patients fully recover, up to 15% remain unwell for 2 or more years. In a primary care study from Seattle, comparing a selective serotonin reuptake inhibitor (SSRI) with a tricyclic antidepressant (TCA), only 50% of patients had fully recovered at 6 months irrespective of initial treatment (Simon *et al.*, 1996). A WHO naturalistic study from 15 centres showed that 60% of those treated with drugs and 50% of milder (untreated cases) were still depressed at 1-year follow up (Goldberg *et al.*, 1998). Outcome is better for recent onset cases. In a sample of over 200 depressed patients drawn from primary care in Manchester, at 4 months 70% of newly diagnosed patients with depression were fully recovered. However, for those patients who had already been treated for depression for more than 3 months, 44% were still unable to continue with their normal lifestyle at a year (Johnson and Mellor, 1977). Even after full recovery, long-term studies indicate that the majority of patients will have a further depressive episode.

WHAT PREDICTS RECOVERY?

Clinical factors
- Recent onset.
- Less severe symptoms.
- Low levels of anxiety.

Social factors
- Current employment.
- No financial difficulties.
- High educational level.
- Reduction in social difficulties or a positive life event.

Interestingly, treatment is a less powerful predictor of outcome than the social and clinical factors listed above, suggesting that social interventions could play a key role in the prevention and management of depression.

Morbidity

Depressive disorders in primary care not only cause considerable personal distress to patients and their families, but also there are marked costs to society (particularly with days off work). In the medical outcomes study from the USA, the level of functioning of community patients with depressive disorders was comparable with, or worse than, that associated with eight other chronic medical conditions, including back problems, arthritis, heart disease and respiratory problems. Depressed patients rated their current health as lower than in all other chronic medical conditions. The number of days spent in bed by patients with depression over the preceding month was only exceeded by patients with current advanced coronary artery disease (Wells *et al.*, 1989). Unsurprisingly, therefore, depressed patients are high utilizers of both primary and secondary healthcare.

RECOGNITION AND DIAGNOSIS

✓ Consultation style.
✓ Screening questions.
✓ Diagnosis.
✓ Diagnostic difficulties.
✓ Risk Assessment.

Although GPs are bound to 'miss' many patients with a depressive disorder, they are more likely to recognize those patients with severe symptoms and social impairment. These are the very patients most likely to respond to treatment. Patients with 'undetected depression' are generally less severely ill and have been ill for a shorter time than patients whose illness has been recognized. Disclosure to the GP of 'undetected depression' does not necessarily improve prognosis, reflecting the fact that the detection of depression in primary care is probably a marker of severity. It is more important that GPs concentrate their efforts on treating well those patients whose depression they do recognize, rather than picking up more, but milder, cases.

Recognition of emotional distress can be enhanced by certain consultation skills:

CONSULTATION STYLE THAT IMPROVES RECOGNITION OF EMOTIONAL DISTRESS

- More eye contact.
- Less avoidant, more relaxed posture.
- Facilitatory noises whilst listening.
- Less urgency at the start.
- Initial use of open questions leading to directive questions about psychosocial issues.
- Do not give information early.

(Tylee, 1999)

Patient factors clearly influence recognition. Many patients normalize or give a somatic explanation to their symptoms – these patients are less likely to be recognized as depressed. Another factor reducing recognition is the tendency to leave mentioning psychosocial problems until late in the consultation.

Screening instruments may aid the recognition of depression in primary care but have not convincingly been shown to influence subsequent recovery. A two-question screen in which a positive test result was a 'yes' to either question, has been shown to have a 96% sensitivity at picking up depression but only a 57% specificity. Hence it will pick up most cases of depression, but has a high rate of false positives.

TWO QUESTIONS TO PICK UP DEPRESSION

- During the last month have you often been bothered by feeling down, depressed or hopeless?
- During the last month have you often been bothered by little interest or pleasure in doing things?

(Whooley *et al.*, 1997)

Diagnosis

If the GP is alerted to the possibility of the presence of a depressive disorder, how then can it quickly and easily be diagnosed? The key depressive symptoms can be grouped into three clusters: mood, biological and cognitive symptoms (Table 1.2).

A useful symptom to distinguish depressive disorders from normal sadness, or simply being fed up, is the presence or absence of anhedonia. Anhedonia is the symptom describing lack of enjoyment from usually pleasurable activities. Patients who are simply feeling fed up will be cheered up when nice things happen to them. However, for those patients suffering from a depressive disorder, not only will they not gain their usual enjoyment from such pleasurable activities, but it may make them feel worse in that it brings home to them the clear change in their mood. Other common symptoms in mild depression include tiredness and reduced concentration.

In the ICD-10 primary care classification of depressive disorders, and in the more widely used American Diagnostic and Statistical Manual of Mental Disorders (DSM-IV), two symptoms are picked out as being of key importance:

- Low or sad mood.
- Loss of interest or pleasure (anhedonia).

Table 1.2. Key diagnostic symptoms

Mood symptoms
Low/depressed mood
Anhedonia (no pleasure in usual activities)

Biological/physical symptoms	*Cognitive symptoms*
Sleep disturbance	Poor concentration
Appetite disturbance	Suicidal/morbid thoughts
Tiredness	Guilt/worthlessness
Psychomotor retardation/agitation	

One of these two key symptoms must be present in a diagnosis of depressive disorder. A variable number of other depressive symptoms may then be added to this. Symptoms of anxiety and nervousness are frequently present. Asking about social impairment will assist in determining the severity of the disorder, which is important in determining the need for treatment. A minimum duration of 2 weeks is usually set to exclude transient stress-related adjustment disorders.

There are three broad categories of patients presenting with depressive disorders in primary care.

DEPRESSIVE DISORDERS IN PRIMARY CARE

Major depression
- Low mood.
- Four or more additional key symptoms.
- Minimum 2-week duration.
- Significant distress or impairment.

Milder depression
- Not meeting criteria for major depression.
- Often recent onset in response to stress.
- Often associated with anxiety symptoms.

Dysthymia
- Chronic (2 years plus) duration.
- Not meeting criteria for major depression.

Making one of these diagnoses has implications for treatment. Major depression is a diagnostic term and can be mild, moderate or severe. Milder depression is sometimes called mixed anxiety and depression.

Diagnostic difficulties

Depression and anxiety

There is a large overlap between depressive disorders and anxiety disorders. In the USA, doctors talk in terms of depressive disorder being co-morbid with generalized anxiety disorder, social phobia, panic disorder and so on. Such distinctions seem to be of little value in primary care where it is clear that anxious and depressive symptoms are part of the same illness process. Few cases of depressive disorder are without associated symptoms of anxiety; similarly, patients with anxiety disorders will often have some associated depressive symptoms.

There is evidence that for patients with both depressive disorders and panic attacks, the course is more chronic, with higher levels of disability and increased suicidality. Similarly, depression and social phobia predicts a poorer outcome. If in doubt as to the main diagnosis, it is probably sensible to diagnose and treat a depressive disorder in the expectation that the anxious symptoms will also resolve.

Excluding a physical diagnosis

A real dilemma in primary care is the extent to which one needs to investigate patients to exclude a physical cause. For example, should the tired patient have a full blood count and thyroid function tests? It is impossible to be completely prescriptive about this. Whether physical investigations are undertaken, and the extent to which they are undertaken, will vary not only with the doctor, but also with a variety of patient factors including the patient's belief about their illness, the way in which symptoms present, previous history and demographic factors.

Diagnosing depression in the physically ill

Poor sleep and poor appetite are common symptoms in physical illness. In research studies amongst physically ill populations, depressive diagnoses are made that have less reliance on these physical symptoms. In primary care, however, it is sensible to be less purist and err on the side of being over-inclusive in the diagnosis and treatment of depression in the physically ill. The evidence overwhelmingly points to under-recognition and under-treatment for this group, despite the effectiveness of usual treatments.

Dysthymia

Dysthymia is a diagnosis little used in primary care, although very common in community samples (with a prevalence rate of approximately 3%). Dysthymia is a chronic depressive illness (2 years or more) of low severity. Depressed mood should have been present for most of the day, and for more days than not, over the 2-year period. It can sometimes be hard to distinguish whether the depressive symptoms are a clear-cut disorder or part of a depressive component in the patient's personality. The importance of dysthymia is that it can be a cause of considerable social morbidity. Drug treatments are effective, in the short term at least, and hence worth trying for those patients with low-grade but chronic symptoms.

RISK ASSESSMENT

Patients with depressive disorders are not only at risk of self-harm, but also have an increased risk of being violent to others. All patients with depressive disorder must be asked about suicidal thoughts. The questions will become more focussed depending on response.

ASKING ABOUT SUICIDE

- Have things got so bad that you don't want to go on?
- Have you actually thought about what you might do?
- Have you taken any steps to put such a plan in place (e.g. buying a hose pipe, making arrangements for the children)?
- How close do you think you are to trying to kill yourself?

Table 1.3. Risk factors for suicide

Clinical risk factors	Relative risk
Recent self-harm	14
Definite plan	5
Hopelessness	3
Severe depressive symptoms	3
Psychotic symptoms (delusions, hallucinations)	3
Alcohol and drug misuse	2
Background risk factors	
1st degree family history of suicide	4
Bereavement	3
Male	1.5
Living alone	1.5
Physical illness	
Recent psychiatric hospital discharge	

(Centre for Evidence Based Mental Health (CEBM) Website)

Certain clinical and demographic factors point to an increased risk of suicide (Table 1.3).

Almost all patients with depressive disorders will have had thoughts of suicide, or at the very least morbid thoughts about death and illness. Many patients immediately add that they have no intention of acting upon such thoughts and have made no plans. A second group of patients have had both suicidal thoughts and also some thoughts about the mechanism of the suicidal act, such as taking an overdose or crashing the car. A third group of patients have started clear planning for a suicide including securing the method by which they intend to kill themselves, making final acts and considering the timing and venue. It is this third group of patients who need an urgent referral to the specialist psychiatric services. In the second group of patients, treatment and regular review with further enquiry about the intensity of their suicidal thoughts might well be appropriate.

An assessment of the risk of violence to others is particularly important if there are children or vulnerable adults. Ask about increased irritability, losing control, and thoughts about harming others.

TREATMENT IN PRIMARY CARE

✓ Who to treat.
✓ How to treat.
✓ How to stop antidepressants.
✓ Mechanism of action of antidepressants.

Who to treat is probably the key question facing the GP – the treatment decision being more important than the diagnostic one. The treatment decision should, however, follow on from the diagnosis made – distinguishing between major depression, milder depression and dysthymia. Amongst the plethora of guidelines on offer for the treatment of depressive disorder, those produced by the British Association for Psychopharmacology (Anderson *et al.*, 2000) are sensible, thorough and evidence based. The treatment recommendations made below draw heavily on these guidelines.

WHO TO TREAT

- Patients with major depression: low mood/anhedonia plus four or more depressive symptoms – duration of 2 or more weeks.
- Patients with milder depression who have been unwell for several weeks and have associated social impairment.
- Patients with physical illness but fewer than four clear psychological symptoms.
- Patients with a more severe illness, irrespective of symptom number and duration.
- Patients with dysthymia.

Acute milder depressions do not clearly benefit from antidepressants. Watchful waiting, education, support and monitoring are as effective as more active treatments. Patients with dysthymia do benefit from antidepressant medication, but there is no evidence for benefit from psychological treatments.

Reactive or endogenous: does it matter?

In the past a distinction was made between those cases of depression which were a response to life's crises (reactive), and those which occurred out of the blue (endogenous). Reactive depression was seen as less severe, understandable and perhaps not requiring medication. Endogenous depression was seen as more severe and needing drug treatment. In fact, most patients are suffering from depressive disorders as a reaction to life's stress. Amongst a group of primary care depressed patients in South West London, over 80% were experiencing social stress (independent of the depression) at the time of presentation (Sireling *et al.*, 1985). Clearly, therefore, most patients seen in primary care are suffering from what would have been called in the past a reactive depression. Treatment outcome does not depend on whether there seems to be an understandable cause for the depression, hence the distinction between reactive and endogenous should be dropped. The decision to treat should not be influenced by whether there is an understandable explanation for the depressive episode.

How to treat

If the patient has a depressive disorder requiring treatment, management can be seen as a series of stages, not all of which need to be completed at the initial consultation. These stages will be for the prescription of anti-depressant medication but the appropriate use of psychological treatments will also be considered.

STAGE ONE: EXPLANATION AND REASSURANCE

- Depression is common.
- There may or may not be an understandable cause.
- Depression is not a sign of weakness.
- Effective treatments are available.

Patients often ask for an explanation as to why they have become depressed, this can be summarized:

- Inherited vulnerability (positive family history in about half of cases).
- Childhood factors resulting in adult vulnerability (death of parent in childhood, abusive experiences).
- Chronic stresses (no close relationships, financial strains, child care problems).
- Precipitating life event (the final straw).

STAGE TWO: DISCUSSION OF TREATMENT OPTIONS

- Drug and psychological treatments are effective.
- If drug treatments are to be used, need to allay patient concerns (see stage 3).
- If psychological treatment to be used, need to ensure effective treatments are available within acceptable time delay.
- Social interventions may be of value if available, e.g. befriending schemes, social activity.

Depressive disorders respond to drug, psychological and social interventions. The reality of general practice, at least in the UK, is that drug treatments are the most readily available option and, if tolerated by the patient, both convenient and effective. Most depressed patients, however, will come to the surgery with a view that counselling is their preferred option. A survey of public opinion conducted by the Royal College of General Practitioners and the Royal College of Psychiatrists found that 90% of the general public thought that the treatment of depression should be counselling compared with only 24% who thought that the treatment should involve antidepressants (Paykel *et al.*, 1998). Therefore, if medication is to be used the GP must offer a clear and careful explanation setting out potential benefits of treatment and allaying concerns.

There are few clinical pointers to assist the choice between drug treatments and talking treatments. Most psychological treatments will usually be given by a specialist, either within the primary care team or from outside. The use of a talking treatment as first line may be appropriate if:

- An appropriate practitioner is available to deliver a treatment known to be effective for depression.
- Patient preference for psychological treatment having been appraised of the options.
- Medication is contraindicated.

The most common treatment used in primary care will be antidepressant medication. In that the depressed patient comes into the surgery primed with concerns about antidepressant medication, it is clearly important that these concerns are allayed or it is unlikely that the patient will adhere to the treatment option provided. Compliance with antidepressant medication is poor with over 50% of patients stopping their medication by 4 weeks. When questioned patients give four main reasons for this:

- Side-effects.
- A belief that pills will not solve their problems.
- A fear of dependence.
- Not being aware of the length of time for which the treatment should be continued.

In order to deal with these very real concerns and misunderstandings, certain key facts need to be given to the patient. These are set out in stage 3.

STAGE THREE: KEY FACTS ABOUT ANTIDEPRESSANTS TO BE SHARED WITH THE PATIENT

■ Antidepressant medication is an effective treatment. If the medication is taken, about two-thirds of patients will be better within 8 weeks.

■ Medication clearly does not resolve social problems but will improve mood and symptoms so that patients then can resolve their problems more effectively.

■ Depressive symptoms may not start to improve for 2–4 weeks. However, depending on the drug chosen, there may be early improvement in some symptoms, e.g. anxiety and poor sleep.

■ Antidepressants are not tranquillizers and do not cause dependence.

■ All drugs have side-effects and antidepressants are no different in this regard, but many side-effects resolve in the first couple of weeks and antidepressants are tolerated well by most patients. If the patient is unable to tolerate the particular drug chosen, there are other drugs with different side-effects that may be more suitable.

Compliance is improved if patients have received the following information (Lin *et al.*, 1995):

■ Take the medication daily.
■ Antidepressants must be taken for 2–4 weeks for a noticeable effect.
■ Continue medication even if feeling better.
■ What to do if you have questions about the medication.
■ Scheduling pleasant activities.

Asking about previous antidepressant experiences and the patient's views about their illness is also associated with better adherence.

Which drug should I choose?

Table 1.4. Currently available antidepressants	
Tricyclics and tricyclic like	*Therapeutic dose*
Amitriptyline	150 mg
Clomipramine	150 mg
Dothiepin	150 mg
Imipramine	150 mg
Lofepramine	140 mg
Trimipramine	150 mg
SSRI	
Citalopram	20 mg
Fluoxetine	20 mg
Fluvoxamine	100 mg
Paroxetine	20 mg
Sertraline	50 mg
Newer antidepressants	
Mirtazapine	30 mg
Nefazodone	200 mg bd
Reboxetine	4 mg bd
Trazodone	150 mg
Venlafaxine	75 mg
MAOI	
Phenelzine	15 mg tds
Moclobemide (a reversible, selective MAOI)	150 mg bd

Approximately 30 antidepressants are now available on prescription in the UK. The newer drugs are no more effective than the older TCAs. All drugs result in recovery or significant improvement in about two-thirds of patients by the end of 8 weeks. Symptomatic improvement occurs first – full restoration of psychosocial functioning may take several months. Such recovery rates are from clinical trials, with reduced compliance in real practice recovery rates are less. The drugs available do differ in their side-effects, toxicity and mechanism of action, and it is probably sensible for each doctor to get to know one or two drugs from each of the main classes of antidepressants available and stick to these.

For convenience currently available antidepressants are listed in four groups, the SSRIs, the TCAs, the monoamine oxidase reuptake inhibitors (MAOIs) and the newer antidepressants (Table 1.4). The table is not exhaustive, but does include those antidepressants that are likely to be prescribed routinely in primary care. There are available some compound preparations of both antidepressants and neuroleptics; there is no reason to prescribe such compounds.

Stage four indicates the factors involved in choosing an antidepressant.

STAGE FOUR: CHOICE OF ANTIDEPRESSANT

- Has the patient had a previous positive response to a particular drug (or family history of a positive response to a drug)?
  - Choose that drug.
- Am I concerned about the patient taking an overdose?
  - If 'yes' avoid TCAs and MAOIs.
- Do I want a sedative drug?
  - Consider: amitriptyline; mirtazapine; trazodone.
- Are there coexisting medical problems?
  - Avoid TCA if cardiac disease, glaucoma, prostatic disease.
  - Avoid cytochrome P450 inhibitors (paroxetine, fluoxetine, fluvoxamine) if the patient is on erythromycin, carbamazepine, ketoconazole, antitubercular drugs.
- Do I want to avoid sexual side-effects?
  - Consider: nefazodone, mirtazapine.
- What will the cost be?

Arguments continue about whether the cheaper TCAs should be used as first-line treatment in the absence of contraindications. Large meta-analyses of trials comparing SSRIs with TCAs indicate that the side-effect profile of the two groups of drugs differs, but this does not necessarily lead to a significantly increased drop out rate for patients on TCAs. The drug cost of the SSRIs is more than the cost of the TCAs. The issue of cost effectiveness and cost benefit, however, is more complex than the simple cost of the tablet. It remains unclear in real practice as opposed to clinical trials whether the simpler dosing regime and the different side-effect profile of the SSRIs results in improved patient outcome or in different total costs. A study in primary care in Seattle (Simon *et al.*, 1996) in which depressed patients were either started on a TCA or an SSRI found that the SSRI was better tolerated than the TCA resulting in better compliance, fewer general practice visits but higher drug costs. However, there was no difference in outcome between the two groups at 6 months with only 50% in each group having recovered. The cost benefit equation is changing as the SSRIs come off patent.

Pragmatically an SSRI is likely to be the first choice if:

- The patient has had a previous good response to the drug.
- There is concern about the risk of overdose.
- The patient is unable or unlikely to tolerate the anticholinergic side-effects of the TCAs.
- A simple once daily regime is likely to aid compliance.
- You wish to avoid sedation.

An SSRI may be avoided if the patient has agitation, marked insomnia or is concerned about sexual dysfunction.

A sedative TCA, such as amitriptyline or clomipramine, may be the first choice if, again, the patient has shown a previous good response to the drug or the patient's symptoms indicate that a sedative antidepressant is likely to help either with insomnia or anxiety. (Table 1.5 gives a comparison of side-effects between SSRIs and TCAs.)

One of the newer antidepressants might be chosen because of its particular side-effect profile.

Which SSRI should I choose?

It is clear that the similarities between the SSRIs greatly outweigh the differences despite the efforts of some pharmaceutical companies to convince us otherwise. There is no convincing evidence that the presence

Table 1.5. Side-effects of SSRIs and TCAs

Adverse effects	SSRI event rates	TCA event rates
Dry mouth	21%	55%
Constipation	10%	22%
Dizziness	13%	23%
Nausea	22%	12%
Diarrhoea	13%	5%
Anxiety	13%	7%
Agitation	14%	8%
Insomnia	12%	7%
Nervousness	15%	11%
Headache	17%	14%

(CEBM Website)

or absence of anxiety symptoms should influence choice of SSRI. Some real differences do exist, however, which may influence prescribing:

- Fluoxetine has a much longer half-life than the other SSRIs. Hence if there is to be a switch to another drug a longer washout period may be needed (6 weeks). However, missed doses are less important and the drug can probably be stopped without a taper period.
- Fluvoxamine, paroxetine and fluoxetine are strong inhibitors of cytochrome P450 enzymes and may raise drug levels of those drugs broken down by this route.
- There is some evidence that fluvoxamine both in clinical trials and in clinical practice is less effective than the other drugs in this group (Depression Guideline Panel, 1993; MacKay *et al.*, 1997).
- Nausea and vomiting are the most frequently reported side-effects for the SSRIs and the main reason for discontinuing treatment. Fluvoxamine is probably the worst drug for this effect.
- Withdrawal events are probably greater with paroxetine compared with the other SSRIs (MacKay *et al.*, 1997).
- Pragmatically, as the SSRIs come off patent, clear price differentials will assist choice.

What dose should I use?

For the SSRIs and the newer antidepressants choosing the dose of medication is easy. Patients are usually started on a once daily therapeutic dose. For the TCAs, the situation is different – these drugs have side-effects that require stepwise increase in dosage. Psychiatric folklore indicates that the treatment dose for the commonly used TCAs (amitriptyline, clomipramine, dothiepin and imipramine) is 150 mg a day. The strength of such evidence is only rated at the level of expert opinion by the Centre of Evidence Based Mental Health. In primary care, patients are often started on doses between 25 mg and 75 mg a day. Doses are then increased slowly, if at all. The question is, how effective are these low doses of TCAs? The evidence supporting the need for the 'therapeutic' doses of TCAs, although clear in psychiatric practice, is much less robust in primary care. The lower doses of TCAs may be effective in treating anxiety symptoms and sleep problems, and this together with placebo and non-specific effects may well be helpful in bringing about a recovery for patients at the milder end of the depression spectrum. A meta-analysis looking at how the dose of antidepressant medication influenced both outcome and side-effects found that low doses of antidepressants were only moderately less effective than higher doses. The low doses were more effective than placebo and caused significantly fewer adverse events (side-effects and drop outs) than the higher doses (Bollini *et al.*, 1999). Hence there is a trade off between a slight reduction in effectiveness and improved tolerance at the lower doses (Table 1.6).

Table 1.6. Antidepressant dose reponse

Dose (mg) imipramine equivalent	Patients showing at least 50% improvement	Adverse event* rate/week
Placebo	35%	0.22
<100	46%	0.22
100–200	53%	0.30
201–250	46%	0.36
250+	48%	0.48

* Side-effects or drop outs   (Bollini *et al.*, 1999)

Follow up

Although direct evidence for the optimum frequency of monitoring of patients on antidepressants is lacking, benefit has been shown for interventions that have included antidepressant drug counselling (Peveler *et al.*, 1999), telephone monitoring (Simon *et al.*, 2000) and weekly psychological contacts (Katon *et al.*, 1996). Early review is needed to monitor response, side-effects and suicide risk.

If the patient is taking the antidepressant and there has been no improvement by 4–6 weeks, response is unlikely by continuing with the same treatment. For patients who responded to a course of fluoxetine by week 8, 55% had started to respond by 2 weeks, 80% by 4 weeks and 90% by 6 weeks. Put another way, the lack of onset of response at 4–6 weeks is associated with a 73–88% chance of no response at 8 weeks (Nierenberg *et al.*, 2000). Elderly patients may take longer to respond to treatment.

STAGE FIVE: FOLLOW UP OF PRESCRIPTION

- Early follow up (1–2 weeks) to check adherence and provide support. Telephone consultation and the use of suitably-trained, non-medical staff may be appropriate.
- If insomnia continues to be a problem, consider a brief course of hypnotic or sedative antidepressant (e.g. trazodone 100 mg).
- If the patient is unable to tolerate the drug, switch to a drug with a different side-effect profile.
- Follow up at 4–5 weeks: if there is no benefit, switch to an antidepressant from a different class. If the response is partial, either wait or increase the dose.

Treatment options if the patient has failed to respond to the initial antidepressant

STAGE SIX: FAILURE TO RESPOND

Non-response at 4–6 weeks
- ?Adequate dose.
- Check compliance.
- Consider social factors.
- Review the diagnosis.

Partial response at 4–6 weeks
- Continue treatment for a further 2 weeks.
- Increase the dose.

Non-response or persisting partial response
- Switch to another class of antidepressant.

Elderly patients
- Consider treatment for up to 9 weeks before changing.

If a patient does not respond to one antidepressant drug, it is comparatively simple to try a preparation with a different mode of action. Although it would seem logical to choose an antidepressant with a different mode of action, there is evidence that simply switching to a different drug in the same class is also effective. When swapping from one antidepressant to another, abrupt withdrawal should usually be avoided. Cross tapering is preferred where the initial drug is slowly reduced over 2–3 weeks and the new drug slowly introduced (Taylor *et al.*, 1999).

If the first-line drug was an SSRI, a second line option would be to either use a TCA, or use one of the newer drugs (reboxetine has a specific effect on noradrenaline (NA) reuptake, venlafaxine and mirtazapine have an effect on both NA and serotonin (5-HT)). If an MAOI is chosen as a second line drug, a suitable washout period needs to be allowed before the MAOI is started. Fluoxetine has a long half-life and hence there needs to be a 6-week washout period before an MAOI can be started, for the TCAs and the other SSRIs a 14-day washout period is needed. Venlafaxine in high dose may be more effective than other antidepressants for treatment-resistant patients.

How long should antidepressants be continued following response?

STAGE SEVEN: CONTINUATION TREATMENT

- Continue antidepressant drug treatment for a minimum of 6 months after remission of major depression, 12 months in the elderly.
- Continue the same dose of antidepressant as used during the acute phase.
- Patients with recurrent major depression should go on to receive maintenance (long-term) antidepressant drug treatment.
- Patients with residual depressive symptoms and other factors increasing the risk of relapse of major depression: continue treatment for longer taking into account the persistence of these factors.

If an antidepressant has been effective, it should be continued for 6 months after recovery before considering a cautious withdrawal. Most relapses occur in the first 4 months in adult patients. There is no difference between the treatment dose of medication and the maintenance dose. Incomplete recovery is the most important risk factor for relapse within the first year of treatment withdrawal. Before withdrawing therapy, therefore, evidence of depressive symptoms should be sought and, if present, treatment should not be stopped.

If the patient's symptoms worsen when medication is discontinued, the medication should be reinstated and an attempt to discontinue deferred for some months.

Some patients have a rapid response to medication (within a few days).

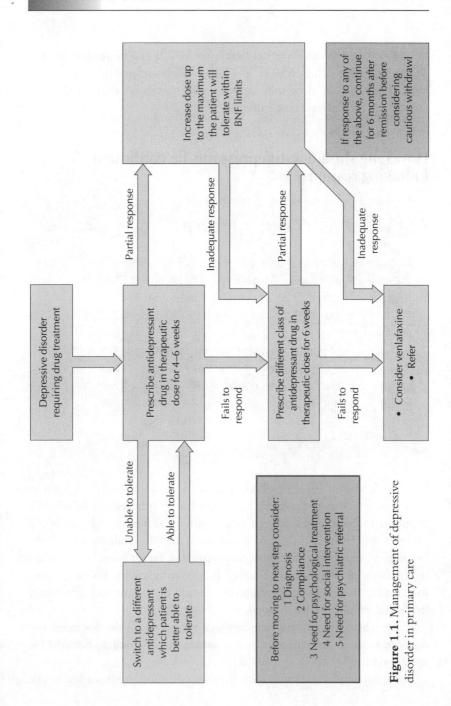

Figure 1.1. Management of depressive disorder in primary care

This is likely to be a placebo response. Such patients do not benefit from a prolonged course of medication and should they remain well, medication can be stopped more quickly.

Figure 1.1 summarizes the drug management of depressive disorder in primary care.

Recurrent depression

Depression is often a chronic disorder and relapse is common, at least 50% after one episode, rising to 90% after three episodes. The relapse rate of depression is reduced by use of long-term maintenance antidepressant medication at full doses. The patient needs to be informed of the risk of relapse and is then able to weigh the balance between this risk and the taking of long-term medication.

How to stop antidepressants

Although patients do not become dependent on antidepressants, patients may experience a discontinuation reaction if the medication is withdrawn too rapidly.

CLINICAL FEATURES OF ANTIDEPRESSANT DISCONTINUATION REACTION

- Abrupt onset within a few days of stopping the antidepressant.
- Symptoms usually resolve within 2 weeks.
- More common following longer courses of treatment.
- Usually mild.
- Rapid resolution with antidepressant reinstatement.

A useful mnemonic is FINISH (Berber, 1998):

Flu-like symptoms, Insomnia, Nausea, Imbalance, Sensory disturbances, Hyperarousal

Table 1.7. Guide to tapering antidepressant doses

Treatment length	Time period during which dosage should be tapered*
6–8 weeks of treatment	3–4 weeks of tapered dosing
4–6 months of treatment	4–8 weeks of tapered dosing
6 months or more of treatment	Reduce dose by one-quarter every 4 weeks

* If dosage is higher than average (for all antidepressants), a longer period of tapering will be needed

The rates of discontinuation symptoms vary with the drug used:

- TCAs: clomipramine probably highest incidence approximately 30%.
- SSRI: incidence varies according to half-life:
  - paroxetine highest (20–60%),
  - fluoxetine lowest (0–14%).
- Others: venlafaxine high rates of discontinuation symptoms reported.

The symptoms of discontinuation can be minimized by gradually tapering the dose (Table 1.7). If symptoms are severe the drug can be reinstated and tapered more gradually. Switching to a drug with a longer half-life, e.g. fluoxetine, may be another option.

How antidepressants work
A basic understanding of the mechanism of action will help choose between the different drugs available.

Mechanism of action of the SSRI
For the SSRIs, the positive benefit and side-effects both result from serotonin action, but on different receptors.

- Benefit: $5-HT_{1a}$ receptor: antidepressant and anxiolytic.
- Side-effects:
  - $5-HT_2$ receptor: agitation/anxiety, akathisia, insomnia, sexual dysfunction (delayed orgasm),
  - $5-HT_3$ receptor: nausea, gastrointestinal problems, headache.

Mechanism of action of TCAs

Whilst the SSRIs have a specific action on the serotonin system, the TCAs exert action on a range of neurotransmitter systems:

- Serotonin (serotonin reuptake inhibitor):
  - benefits and side-effects as explained for the SSRIs.
- Noradrenaline:
  - benefit: antidepressant,
  - side-effects (alpha$_1$ antagonist): hypotension, retrograde ejaculation.
- Acetylcholine:
  - side-effects: constipation, blurred vision, dry mouth, urinary retention.
- Histamine:
  - side-effects: weight gain, drowsiness.

The different TCAs have different selectivity for these neurotransmitter systems. Clomipramine is a powerful inhibitor of 5-HT reuptake with little effect on NA, although there is a marked anticholinergic and antihistaminic effect. Amitriptyline by contrast blocks the reuptake of both 5-HT and NA to a similar degree and also has an anticholinergic and antihistaminic effect. Lofepramine has a largely noradrenergic reuptake blocking effect with little effect on the 5-HT system, together with a reduced anticholinergic and antihistaminic effect compared with the older TCAs.

Mechanism of action of newer antidepressants

The mechanism of action of the newer antidepressants are shown in Table 1.8.

Table 1.8. Mechanism of action of antidepressants

Venlafaxine (serotonin and NA reuptake inhibitor)
Blocks reuptake 5-HT (low doses)
Blocks reuptake 5-HT and NA (moderate and high doses)
No anticholinergic action
No antihistamine action

Mirtazapine (NA and serotonergic antidepressant)
Increases NA and 5-HT release
Blocks $5-HT_2$ receptors (no sexual dysfunction)
Blocks $5-HT_3$ receptors (no gastrointestinal dysfunction)
Antihistamine action (sedative)

Nefazodone
Blocks reuptake 5-HT
Blocks $5-HT_2$ receptor (no sexual dysfunction)

Trazodone
Blocks reuptake 5-HT
Blocks $5-HT_2$ receptor (no sexual dysfunction)
Antihistamine action (sedative)
$Alpha_1$ antagonism (hypotension)

Reboxetine (specific NA reuptake inhibitor)
Blocks NA reuptake
No effect on 5-HT
No anticholinergic action
No antihistamine action

Mechanism of action of MAOIs

The older MAOIs irreversibly block the enzyme monoamine oxidase (MAO) which breaks down 5-HT and NA. Dietary restrictions and drug interactions have limited their use in primary care. Moclobemide is a reversible, selective inhibitor of MAO which does not require dietary restrictions.

PSYCHOLOGICAL TREATMENTS FOR DEPRESSION

✓ Activity scheduling.
✓ Problem-solving treatment.
✓ Counselling.

Specific psychological treatments are known to be as effective as medication for major depression of moderate severity or less. Within primary care there is a range of non-specific and specific psychological interventions that may be available.

The evidence for specific psychological treatments (as with medication) supports treatment for patients with major depression. There is little evidence supporting the use of psychological treatments for patients with dysthymia. For patients with milder depression, encouragement and support would be the first-line psychological intervention, with more specific treatments being reserved for those who do not respond with time and watchful waiting.

When considering a psychological treatment as the sole treatment for a depressive disorder, the following principles apply:

■ Time-limited treatment should be offered focussing on current problems and aiming at symptom reduction rather than personality change.
■ The therapist should be skilled in providing treatment to patients with depression.
■ Symptomatic response should be monitored and medication considered for patients failing to show any improvement by 6–8 weeks or nearly full remission by 12 weeks.

Positive support and encouragement

Humanity and common sense indicate that a patient with depression should be treated in a supportive and encouraging way. It is important to emphasize that by and large patients with depressive disorders do recover with the effective treatments that are available. It is also important to inform patients how common depression is, explaining that many people put on a social façade when they are depressed and it is only family and friends who know the true situation. It is helpful to counter any ideas of depression being a result of weakness or lack of moral fibre.

Behavioural treatments

Patients with depression have usually curtailed social and other activities. They lack the motivation to participate in previously enjoyable activities and have experienced not enjoying such activities even if they have made the effort. A simple and easily understood vicious circle is then set up whereby low mood leads to reduced participation in enjoyable activities further lowering mood (Figure 1.2).

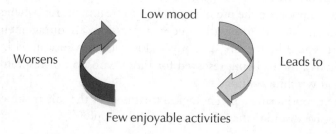

Low mood

Worsens   Leads to

Few enjoyable activities

Figure 1.2. Circle of mood.

ACTIVITY SCHEDULING

- Explain that low mood leads to doing few pleasurable activities.
- Set a goal for a daily, pleasurable, achievable activity – 'a treat a day'.
- Pleasurable tasks to be set by the patient and done even if their motivation is low.
- Include exercise and activities with other people.

Activity scheduling is an effective, simple intervention for depressed patients that points out the vicious circle described above and helps the patient increase pleasurable activities. In essence, the patient must increase the number of pleasurable activities that they participate in whilst, at the same time, if possible, reducing the number of unpleasant activities.

A simple activity prescription can be to ask the patient to engage in either one pleasurable activity a day (a treat a day) or, if this seems too demanding, three or four pleasurable activities a week. It is important to allow the patient to decide for themselves which activities they wish to participate in and to organize the activities for themselves. This planning and organization can help counter the feelings of helplessness felt by many depressed patients. Exercise might not only be an enjoyable activity but also might have beneficial effects in its own right. There is some evidence that participating in aerobic activity lifts mood. Some GPs are able to 'prescribe' sessions at a local gym or leisure centre.

Problem-solving treatment

Problem-solving is a relatively simple psychological treatment based on the following premises:

- The patient's symptoms are caused by practical problems they are facing in everyday life.
- If the patient's problems can be resolved, their symptoms will improve.
- Problems can be resolved through the technique of problem-solving.

Problem-solving treatment over six sessions, given either by a GP or a practice nurse, has been shown to be an effective treatment for major depression and. indeed, as effective as antidepressant medication (Mynors-Wallis *et al.*, 1995, 2000).

Table 1.9 shows that problem–solving is broken down into seven stages.
As with planning simple behavioural treatments, assisting patients in
solving their own problems provides patients with a sense of purpose, and
mastery over their difficulties. Although the full problem–solving treatment is unlikely to be possible within a normal consultation, it can be
helpful to ask patients to identify possible problems and seek solutions to
them.

Table 1.9. Summary of problem-solving treatment

Stage 1: Explanation of the treatment and its rationale

Stage 2: Clarification and definition of problems
Listing the problems in a clear and concrete form and breaking down
large problems into smaller and more manageable parts

Stage 3: Choice of achievable goals
Specific goals are set to be achieved both quickly (before the next
treatment session), and more slowly (over the course of treatment).
Goals should be SMART:
    Specific, Measurable, Achievable, Relevant, Timed

Stage 4: Generating solutions
Consider any relevant solutions to achieve the goals set (brainstorming)

Stage 5: Choice of preferred solution
Consider the pros and cons

Stage 6: Implementation of the preferred solution
Any steps required to implement the preferred solution should be listed
clearly and precisely. The therapist and patient should agree homework
tasks for the patient to carry out before the next session

Stage 7: Evaluation
The patient and therapist evaluate the patient's success or lack of
success in the assigned homework tasks

CASE STUDY: DAVE

Dave is a 42-year-old health service manager, married with two children aged 10 and 12. He rarely attends the surgery, but has come to see Dr Jones complaining of sleeping problems and neck ache. On further questioning Dr Jones discovers that he is under considerable pressure at work with an unsupportive boss and a workload which involves him often not getting home until 7 pm. Dave reports that over the last month he has been increasingly tired and has had poor concentration. He is very reluctant to take medication and so a problem-solving approach is considered.

Dave is asked to list the main problems that he faces. He comes up with two, work as already described and also marital difficulties. He and his wife, Carol, have been arguing a lot recently and have not had sexual intercourse for the past 3 months. Dave admits to being irritable with both Carol and the children; over the past month he has slept in the spare room.

Dr Jones decides to give Dave a sick note for a week to relieve him from the immediate pressure of his job. Dave then chooses his relationship with Carol as the problem he would like to work on over the next week. Dave says that he wants to have a better relationship with his wife. This is turned into a SMART goal of going out for a meal with his wife on one occasion during the next week. Dave discusses how he will broach the subject of his depression with his wife and the plan for going out for a meal. He seems to have a sensible plan and Dr Jones arranges to see him in a week's time.

A week later, Dave has successfully achieved the task of going out to the local Indian restaurant with his wife. Rather to his surprise they had an enjoyable evening. Carol was supportive when Dave told her about the diagnosis of depression. They have decided to go out one evening a week and get Carol's mum to babysit.

Dave remains concerned about his job at work and does not yet feel ready to return. Dr Jones gives him a further week's sick note and asks him to come up with one or two achievable goals concerning his work. At the next appointment, a week later, Dave has identified two particular problems: firstly, the lack of secretarial support and, secondly, the difficult relationship with his immediate boss. He does not feel that he is going to be able to change the relationship with his boss but does think that he could get extra secretarial help if he speaks to the Finance Director on his return to work. He decides that he will return to work making an appointment to see the Finance Director at the earliest opportunity.

Dr Jones does not see Dave again for a further 6 months when he comes with a tennis elbow. Dr Jones finds out that the discussion with the Finance Director led to a more wide-ranging discussion than simply secretarial support. Dave has moved sideways within the organization to a job working with a line manager whom he finds more congenial. He reports having no further depressive symptoms.

Lessons from the case study

- Presentation with somatic symptoms.
- Depression is associated with life stresses.
- Setting achievable goals for problems.
- Patient choice of problems and goals.
- Early success motivates the patient.
- Once started, the patient can continue the process.

Counselling

The British Association for Counselling describes counselling as the skilled and principled use of relationships to develop self-knowledge, emotional acceptance and growth and personal resources. The overall aim is to live more fully and satisfyingly. Counselling may be concerned with addressing and resolving specific problems, making decisions, coping with crises, working through feelings or inner conflict or improving relationships with others. Counselling techniques that focus on current problems rather than past difficulties are more likely to be helpful.

Evidence supporting the use of counselling for patients with depressive disorders is increasing (Roland *et al.*, 2001). Patients like counselling and counselling may be supportive for GPs in the care of their patients. The best evidence as to the place of counselling as a treatment for depression is from three UK studies. The first from North London and Manchester compared cognitive behavioural therapy (CBT), counselling and treatment as usual by the GP, for patients with anxiety and depression (Ward *et al.*, 2000). Both CBT and counselling were more effective than GP usual treatment at 4 months, but no differences were found at a year. A second study from the Midlands (Bedi *et al.*, 2000) found no difference at 8 weeks between counselling and antidepressant medication for patients with major depression, whether or not patients had been randomized or had chosen their treatment. The most recent study (Chilvers *et al.*, 2001) found generic counselling to be as effective as antidepressant medication at 12 months for the treatment of major depression in primary care. Patients recovered more quickly with medication.

There is also evidence that counselling by health visitors is effective for post-natal depression (see Chapter 9).

Although patient satisfaction with counselling is often high, counselling is not free from side-effects. In many areas long delays will leave patients untreated. Treatment approaches that look into past difficulties may make depressed patients feel worse.

Combination treatments

Drug and psychological interventions are not an either/or option. Although there is little evidence that the combination of a specific course of psychological treatment and medication offers benefits over each treatment alone, few drug treatments are given in primary care without at least some supportive comments. A US study looked at whether GPs used specific cognitive behavioural interventions in their consultations with depressed patients, by contacting the depressed patient by telephone at 1 month. Up to 40% of patients reported psychological recommendations, such as planning pleasurable activities, problem-solving and challenging depressive thoughts. Patients not only reported taking this advice, but also it was associated with better adherence to the recommended drug treatment (Robinson *et al.*, 1995).

Other treatments (Geddes et al., 2001)

Herbal treatments

St John's Wort may be an effective herbal remedy for milder depression. It is not a licensed drug and hence dose and purity of preparations may be uncertain. Patients should be warned about drug interactions, particularly with SSRIs.

Exercise

There is some evidence that exercise may be effective – alone or together with other treatments.

Bibliotherapy

There is limited evidence that advising patients to read self-help books, such as *Feeling Good* by David Burns, helps to improve mild depressive symptoms.

Social interventions

A befriending service has been shown to be helpful to some women with chronic depression. Other social interventions are probably effective but have not been evaluated and may be difficult to access from primary care.

DEPRESSION AND PHYSICAL ILLNESS

Physical illness

Antidepressants are effective in the treatment of depression in patients who also have a physical illness (Gill and Hatcher, 1999).

Cardiovascular disease

The concept of dying from a broken heart suggests that popular culture has long known of the link between psychological disorders and cardiovascular disease. The nature of this link is complex:

- Depression is associated with an increased risk of having a myocardial infarction.
- Depressive disorders occur in about 20% of patients admitted with an acute myocardial infarction.
- The presence of a depressive disorder immediately post-myocardial infarction increases the risk of mortality approximately four fold.

In treating patients with depression and cardiovascular disease, the following points should be borne in mind:

- Drug treatment of depressive disorder in the presence of cardiovascular disease should not include the TCAs because of their anticholinergic and antiadrenergic effects. Sertraline and citalopram have the least potential for drug interactions of the SSRIs.
- There is little evidence that psychosocial interventions are of value as part of post-myocardial infarction follow up.
- Patients with non-specific chest pain do benefit from specialist cognitive behavioural therapy.

Cancer

The presence of depression amongst cancer patients varies with the type of malignancy (McDaniel *et al.*, 1995) (Figure 1.3).

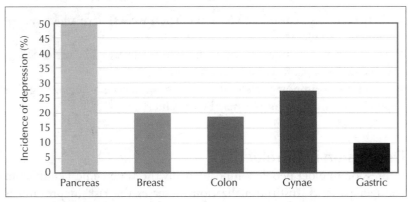

Figure 1.3. Incidence of depression in cancer patients.

Overall about 25% of patients with cancer can be diagnosed as suffering from a depressive disorder with about a similar proportion suffering from anxiety and adjustment disorders.

Depression is under-diagnosed in cancer patients. One difficulty in making the diagnosis is the overlap of physical and psychological symptoms, in particular, fatigue and anorexia. In that there is evidence that medically ill patients may show significant benefit from antidepressant medication even without a full depressive syndrome, it is sensible to err on the side of over-inclusion and, if in doubt, offer a trial of treatment. Consider a drug which avoids gastrointestinal side-effects, e.g. mirtazapine, reboxetine.

- Antidepressant medication improves both symptoms and quality of life in depressed cancer patients
- Individual and group supportive psychosocial interventions have been shown to improve survival times.

Stroke

Post-stroke depression occurs in about 20% of cases drawn from community samples. It is associated with younger age, greater physical and social impairment, cognitive impairment and previous psychiatric history.

The mean duration of a depressive episode is about 9 months, most cases resolving within a year. The presence of depression is associated with increased morbidity.

- Early depressive episodes (within the first 6 weeks) have a high rate of spontaneous recovery.
- Treatment with antidepressant medication is effective. The use of SSRIs is associated with fewer side-effects than TCAs.
- Good social support is associated with good recovery suggesting that psychosocial interventions may be of value.

Depression in the elderly

Depression in older people is fundamentally the same clinical entity as in younger patients. Institutionalization increases the risk (depression is

Table 1.10. Four point Geriatric Depression Scale		
	Score 1	*Score 0*
Are you basically satisfied with your life?	No	Yes
Do you feel your life is empty?	Yes	No
Are you afraid that something bad is going to happen to you?	Yes	No
Do you feel happy most of the time?	No	Yes

Scores of more than 1 are suggestive of depression
Diagnosis must then be made clinically

(Consensus Guidelines, 1999)

present in nearly 50% of nursing-home patients), and there is a strong association with dementia, strokes and Parkinson's disease.

The four point Geriatric Depression Scale may be used to screen patients (Table 1.10).

WHEN TO REFER

- Concern about suicide risk.
- Risk to vulnerable others.
- Psychotic and agitated depression.
- Patients who have not responded to two courses of antidepressant medication.
- Patients with bipolar depression.
- Specific psychological treatment.

Concern about suicide risk

Specialist mental health services play an important role in helping primary care in the assessment and management of patients at risk of suicide.

Risk to vulnerable others

Patients with depressive disorders have increased irritability. If this is the case and there are children and vulnerable adults who might be at risk, referral for advice and support from the Community Mental Health Team (CMHT) might be appropriate.

Psychotic and agitated depression

Any patient whose symptoms give cause for concern that they might have become psychotic should be given an urgent referral. Patients are at risk of self-harm or harm to others. Patients with psychotic depression will need antipsychotic drugs in addition to antidepressants. Patients (often elderly) with an agitated depression may be helped by the increased support and monitoring that can be provided by a CMHT.

Patients who have not responded to two courses of antidepressant medication

These patients will have been treated within primary care for at least a 3–month period before this situation is reached. It might be appropriate to consider a third class of antidepressant medication. However, a psychiatric opinion might be helpful to consider lithium augmentation, or a specialist psychological treatment or psychosocial support from the CMHT.

Patients with bipolar depression

Patients who have had a manic episode are at risk of a switch to mania with antidepressant treatment.

Specific psychological treatment

Local arrangements will dictate how to access specific psychological treatments.

THE ORGANIZATION OF SERVICES FOR PATIENTS WITH DEPRESSION

There is now a considerable body of research, largely from the USA, showing that the outcome for patients with depression in primary care can be improved by altering service delivery. The following have been shown to make a significant improvement in recovery rates:

- Population-based clinical information system.
- Systematic follow up with monitoring of adherence and outcome:
  - telephone contact,
  - regular review appointments,
  - adherence to clinical guidelines.
- Health staff trained in medication management and brief psychological treatments.

The costs of such interventions are offset by the improved recovery rates achieved. Kendrick (2000) recommends that the treatment of depression in primary care should parallel that of other chronic diseases, e.g. diabetes and asthma, with the establishment of nurse-led clinics.

WHAT TO EXPECT FROM SPECIALIST CARE

The treatment of depressive disorders that have not resolved in primary care is the bread and butter of psychiatric practice. An expertise in the pharmacological management of treatment-resistant depression should be available together with access to psychosocial interventions.

In an ideal service, there would be shared guidelines between primary and secondary care for the treatment of depression. Such guidance would include appropriate treatments in both settings and when referral between the two services should occur.

Treatment-resistant drug strategies for depression

Lithium augmentation

Adding lithium to another antidepressant is effective in about 50% of cases of treatment resistant depression.

High-dose venlafaxine

High doses of venlafaxine have been shown to be of value in treatment resistant depression. The dose may be limited by raised blood pressure and increased serotonergic side-effects.

Use of MAOIs

MAOIs are rarely used in primary care but may have a particular role in atypical depression:

ATYPICAL DEPRESSION

- Mood reactivity (i.e. mood brightens in response to positive events).
- Two or more of:
  - weight gain or increase in appetite,
  - increase in sleep,
  - leaden paralysis in limbs,
  - sensitivity to interpersonal rejection.

The combination of MAOIs with some TCAs (not clomipramine) is also used for treatment-resistant depression.

ECT

ECT continues to have a role in the management of severe depressive disorders and is usually given as an inpatient.

Specialist psychological treatments

Cognitive therapy

Cognitive therapy is based on the theoretical rationale that low mood is secondary to 'depressive cognitions'. Systematic errors of thinking are identified. These errors of thinking are underpinned by a set of faulty assumptions based on past experience, e.g. 'Unless I do everything perfectly, I am a failure'.

COGNITIVE ERRORS IN THINKING

- Selective attention to the negative features of a situation.
- Thinking in extremes: magnification of the catastrophic implications of these situations.
- Arbitrary inference: drawing a conclusion for which is there is little or no evidence.
- Over-generalization: drawing a general conclusion on the basis of a single incident.
- Personalization relating external events to oneself in an unwarranted way.
- Dichotomous thinking: seeing everything as black or white.

Treatment is typically 15–20 structured sessions attempting to detect and counter these faulty assumptions and errors in thinking. Treatment is an active collaborative process that tests out assumptions and beliefs in real-life experiences, rather than by persuasion or debate. Cognitive therapy has a behavioural component (activity scheduling and empirical testing of beliefs) – hence treatment should be more precisely termed 'cognitive behavioural therapy'.

GPs may use cognitive strategies during a consultation, e.g. when a patient says, 'It's all my fault, I never seem to get anything right', the response, 'This is how you feel when depressed', or pointing out past successes, are both ways of countering cognitive distortions.

Interpersonal psychotherapy

The rationale underpinning interpersonal psychotherapy is that depression occurs in the context of, if not actually caused by, relationship and social difficulties. If difficulties in these areas are satisfactorily dealt with, the symptoms of depression will resolve. Interpersonal psychotherapy emphasizes the importance of the psychosocial environment in understanding psychiatric disorders. These ideas have been given empirical support by work implicating life events in the aetiology of depression. Stressful life events are often of a psychosocial nature, e.g. marital disharmony and bereavement. Furthermore, depressed patients have impaired social functioning which improves with symptomatic recovery.

Interpersonal psychotherapy is a time-limited (12–16 weeks) psychological treatment which begins by describing the symptoms of depression and explaining that they are understandable and likely to resolve. Interpersonal psychotherapy, like cognitive therapy, deals with events in the present rather than the past. The aims of treatment are of clarification and resolution of one of more of the following interpersonal difficulties:

- Prolonged grief reaction.
- Role disputes.
- Role transitions.
- Interpersonal deficits.

REFERENCES

Anderson IM, Nutt DJ, Deakin FW (2000). Evidence based guidelines for treating depressive disorders with antidepressants. *Journal of Psychopharmacology* **43**:220.

Bedi N, Chilvers C, Churchill R, Dewey M, Duggan C *et al.* (2000) Assessing effectiveness of treatment of depression in primary care partially randomised preference trial. *British Journal of Psychiatry* **177**:317–319.

Berber MJ (1998). Finish remembering the discontinuation syndrome. *Journal of Clinical Psychiatry* **59**:255.

Chilvers C, Dewey M, Fielding K *et al.* (2001). Antidepressant drugs and generic counselling for treatment of major depression in primary care. *British Medical Journal* **332**:772–775.

Consensus Guidelines (1999). *Health and Ageing Guidelines for Depression.* Wyeth, Guildford.

Depression Guideline Panel (1993). *Depression in Primary Care: Volume 1, Detection and Diagnosis Clinical Practice Guideline No. 5.* Rockville MD. US Department of Health and Human Services.

Geddes J, Butler R, Warner J (2001). *Depressive disorders in Clinical Evidence.* Issue 4. BMJ Publishing Group, London.

Gill D, Hatcher S (1999). A systematic review of the treatment with depression with antidepressant drugs in patients who also have a physical illness. *Journal of Psychosomatic Research* **47**:131–43.

Goldberg D, Privett M, Ustun B, Simon G, Linden M (1998). The effects of detection and treatment on the outcome of major depression in primary care. *British Journal of General Practice* **48**:1840–44.

Johnson DAW, Mellor V (1977). The severity of depression in patients treated in general practice. *Journal of the Royal College of General Practitioners* **27**:419–22.

Katon W, Schulberg H (1992). Epidemiology of depression on primary care. *General Hospital Psychiatry* **14**:237–47.

Katon W, Robinson P, Von Korff M, Lin E, Bush T, Ludman E (1996). A multifaceted intervention to improve treatment of depression in primary care. *Archives of General Psychiatry* **53**:924–32.

Kendrick A (2000). Depression management clinics in general practice. *British Medical Journal* **320**:527–8.

Lin E, Von Korff M, Katon W, Bush T, Simon G, Walker E, Robinson P (1995). The role of the primary care physician in patients' adherence to antidepressant therapy. *Medical Care* **33**:67–74.

McDaniel JS, Mussleman DL, Porter MR, Reed DA, Numeroff CB (1995). Depression in patients with cancer. *Archives of General Psychiatry* **52**:89–99.

Mackay FJ, Dunn NR, Wilton LV, Pearce GL, Freemantle SN, Mann RD (1997). A comparison of fluvoxamine, fluoxetine, sertaline and paroxetine examined by observational cohort studies. *Pharmacoepidemiology and Drug Safety* 6235–46.

Mynors-Wallis LM, Gath DH, Lloyd-Thomas AR, Tomlinson D (1995). Randomised controlled trial comparing problem-solving treatment with amitriptyline and placebo for major depression in primary care. *British Medical Journal* **310**:441–5.

Mynors-Wallis LM, Gath DH, Day A, Baker FA (2000). Randomised controlled trial of problem-solving treatment, antidepressant medication and combined treatment for major depression in primary care. *British Medical Journal* **320**:26–31.

Nierenberg AA, Farabaugh AH, Alpert JE, Gordon J, Worthington JJ, Rosenbaum JF, Fava M (2000). Timing of onset of antidepressant response with Fluoxetine treatment. *American Journal of Psychiatry* **157**:1423–8.

Paykel ES, Hart D, Priest RG (1998). Changes in public attitudes to depression during the Defeat Depression Campaign. *British Journal of Psychiatry* **173**:519–22.

Peveler R, George C, Kinmouth AL, Campbell M, Thompson C (1999). Effective antidepressant drug counselling information leaflets on adherence to drug treatment in primary care. *British Medical Journal* **319**:612–15.

Robinson P, Bush T, Von Korff M, Katon W, Lin E, Simon GE, Walker E (1995). Primary care physician use of cognitive behavioural techniques with depressed patients. *Journal of Family Practice* **4**:352–7.

Roland N, Bauer P, Mellerclark J, Hayward P, Godfrey C (2001). Counselling for depression in primary care. *Cochrane Review in Cochrane Library Issue 1*, 2001. Oxford.

Simon GE, Von Korff M, Heilgenstein JH, Revicki DA, Grothaus L, Katon W, Wager EH (1996). Initial antidepressant choice in primary care: Effectiveness and cost of fluoxetine versus tricyclic antidepressants. *Journal of the American Medical Association* **275**:897–902.

Simon GE, Von Korff M, Rutter C, Wagner E (2000). Randomised trial of monitoring feedback and management of care by telephone to improve treatment of depression in primary care. *British Medical Journal* **320**:550-554.

Sireling LI, Frieling P, Paykel ES, Rao BM (1985). Depression in general practice. Clinical features and comparison with out-patients. *British Journal of Psychiatry* **147**:119–26.

Taylor D, McConnell D, McConnell H, Abel K, Kerwin R (1999). *The Maudsley Prescribing Guidelines*, 5th edition. Martin Dunitz, London.

Tylee A (1999). Depression in the community: physician and patient perspective. *Journal of Clinical Psychiatry* **60 (Supl 7)**:12–18.

Ward E, King M, Lloyd M, Bauer P, Sibbald B, Farrerly S, Gabbay M, Tarrier N, Addington, Hall J (2000). Randomised controlled trial of non-directive counselling, cognitive behaviour therapy and usual general practitioner care for patients with depression. *British Medical Journal* **321**:13838.

Wells KB, Stewart A, Hayes RD *et al.* (1989). The functioning and wellbeing of depressed patients. Results and medical outcome study. *Journal of the American Medical Association* **262**:914–19.

Whooley MA, Avins AL, Mirander J, Browner WS (1997). Case finding instruments for depression. Two questions are as good as many. *Journal of General and International Medicine* **12**:439–45.

FURTHER READING

Burns D (1980). *Feeling Good: the New Mood Therapy*. New American Library, New York.

Stahl S (1997). *Psychopharmacology of Antidepressants*. Martin Dunitz, London.

WEBSITES

Centre for Evidence Based Mental Health
http://cebmh.warn.ox.ac.uk/cebmh/frames.html
Guidelines for the management of depression in primary care.

Depression Central
www.psycom.net/depression.central.html
Information on all types of depressive disorders and treatments.

SELF-HELP

Depression Alliance
35 Westminster Bridge Road, PO Box 1022, London 7QB
Tel: 020 7633 0557
Website: www.depressionalliance.org
A charity run by people who have personally suffered from depression.

Fellowship of Depressives Anonymous
36 Chestnut Avenue, Beverly HU17 9QU
Tel: 01482 860619
Website: www.ribblewebdesign.co.uk
Offers self-help for depressives, their friends and families and provides support and advice for setting up groups.

Manic Depression Fellowship
8–10 High Street, Kingston-on-Thames KT1 1EY
Tel: 020 8974 6550
Provides support, advice and information for people with manic depression, their families, friends and carers.

Manic Depression Fellowship (Scotland)
7 Woodside Crescent, Glasgow G37 UL
Tel: 0141 331 0344

Provides support, advice and information for people with manic depression, their families, friends and carers.

Manic Depression Fellowship (Wales)
Belmont, St Cadoc's Hospital, Caerleon, Newport NP6 1XQ
Tel: 01633 430430
Provides support, advice and information for people with manic depression, their families, friends and carers.

MIND – National Association for Mental Health
Granta House, 15–19 Broadway, Stratford, London E15 4BQ
Tel: 020 8519 2122 (admininstration)
        0345 660163 (information line)
Provides support for people in mental distress and their families. Advice, campaigns and local services. Legal advice. More than 200 local groups in England and Wales.

Scottish Association for Mental Health
Atlantic House, 38 Gardner's Crescent, Edinburgh EH3 8DQ
Tel: 0131 229 9687
Independent voluntary organization dealing with all aspects of mental illness and health in Scotland.

The Samaritans
10 The Grove, Slough SL1 1QQ
Tel: 01753 216500 (administration)
        0345 909090 (nationwide helpline)
Website: www.samaritans.org.uk
Offers confidential support 24 hours a day to those in emotional crisis.

Seasonal Affective Disorder Association
P O Box 989, Steyning, Sussex BN44 3HG
Tel: 01903 814942
Fax: 01903 814942
Provides advice to sufferers.

Mental Health Helpline
Tel: 0345 660606
A 24-hour national helpline for information and support.

chapter 2

The anxious patient

IN THIS CHAPTER

- How to explain anxiety disorders to patients.
- Physical and psychological disorders to exclude.
- How to treat anxiety disorders with brief, simple psychological interventions.
- How to treat anxiety disorders with medication.
- Obsessive compulsive disorder; post-traumatic stress disorder.
- When and where to refer.

INTRODUCTION

Fear is an emotion understood by most people. When we are fearful we usually have a good idea of what is making us feel scared. We have some understanding of the physical symptoms and can also understand our behaviour. Anxiety, which may produce an almost identical physiological and behavioural reaction, is often not understood. An individual may either not be able to identify a 'threat', or they may realize that their reaction to a perceived threat is irrational or exaggerated. To fill this gap in understanding, individuals may make sense of what is happening by concluding that they have a serious physical illness or that they are on the verge of losing control and are about to become seriously mentally ill. Perhaps the most important skill for a GP helping a patient with an anxiety disorder is the ability to listen, reassure and help fill the 'gap in understanding'.

Table 2.1. Epidemiology of anxiety disorders

Number of patients on the average GP's list: 400

Lifetime prevalence: 25%

Risk factors: women x2, family history, stressful event

Associated conditions: depression, alcohol abuse

EPIDEMIOLOGY

Anxiety disorders are very common. A UK community survey found that 10% of women and 5% of men were suffering from a non-specific neurotic disorder in the week of the survey (Meltzer *et al.*, 1995). Generalized anxiety disorder was found in 3.4% of women and 2.8% of men and panic disorder in just under 1% of both men and women. Many individuals with less severe anxiety disorders never seek medical help; however, there will be a significant number of patients on any GP's list whose lives are severely curtailed by anxiety disorders (Table 2.1).

Although anxiety disorders are often seen as being at the milder end of the psychiatric disorders, their prevalence and chronicity mean they have a marked impact on social functioning, and a greater public health impact in terms of disability adjusted years than AIDS or many cancers.

The course of anxiety disorders tends to be chronic. In one study, it was estimated that 80% of patients with a generalized anxiety disorder will have the disorder 3 years later. Those patients with anxiety disorders persisting for more than a year will be frequent attenders (>12 visits per year) over the next 10 years (Lloyd *et al.*, 1996).

RECOGNITION AND DIAGNOSIS

The key features of anxiety disorders are marked feelings of fear, worry and apprehension, which are excessive in the context of any potential threat. Many patients will present not with anxiety, but with a number of physical symptoms. Panic attacks may be a feature, when patients experience rapidly escalating symptoms of anxiety and often believe they will lose control or suffer a major physical illness. Hyperventilation may also be present with anxiety disorders and can sometimes be responsible for a number of the anxious symptoms.

Symptoms present in anxiety disorders can be grouped as psychological, physical and behavioural (Table 2.2).

Table 2.2. Common symptoms in anxiety disorders

Psychological
Anticipatory fear
Excessive worry
Restlessness, feeling on edge, keyed up
Difficulty concentrating
Irritability
Tiredness, easily fatigued

Physical
Gastrointestinal: dry mouth or difficulty swallowing; diarrhoea; excess wind; abdominal discomfort
Genitourinary: frequency/urgency micturition; menstrual pain/disturbance; erectile dysfunction
Neuromuscular: aching muscles including chest pain, headaches, tremor, shaking, tingling sensations
Cardiovascular: palpitations, pounding heart; dizziness
Respiratory: hyperventilation; difficulty inhaling, feeling short of breath
Other features: sleep disturbance; derealization/depersonalization; sweating

Behavioural
Avoidance of feared situations
Rituals to reduce anxiety (obsessive compulsive disorder (OCD))

The dilemma for the GP in the presence of anxious symptoms is the need to exclude some alternative diagnoses yet at the same time not to arrange an array of tests which may worsen an individual's anxiety or tendency towards somatization. Appropriate history taking, examination and, if necessary, investigations are not only part of making a diagnosis of an anxiety disorder, but may also provide appropriate reassurance for the patient.

Differential diagnosis of anxiety

Physical illnesses which may mimic anxiety disorders are listed below. A physical cause is less likely if there is a clear psychological explanation for the anxiety, the anxiety is situation specific or there is a premorbid history of anxiety or depression. A physical cause is more likely if there are episodic symptoms without an obvious psychological cause.

Physical disorders which may be mistaken for anxiety disorders

- Thyrotoxicosis.
- Hypoglycaemia.
- Tachyarrhythmias.
- Menière's syndrome.
- Phaeochromocytoma.
- Addison's disease.

PSYCHOLOGICAL DISORDERS WHICH MAY BE MISTAKEN FOR ANXIETY

- Depression and anxiety commonly coexist: do not mistake agitated depression for anxiety.
- Schizophrenia: fear may be the result of delusional thinking or hallucinations. A feeling of unease may precede frank psychotic symptoms.
- Substance abuse: withdrawal symptoms, self-medication.
- Dementia.

It is not only physical illness that may be mistaken for anxiety, many forms of psychological illness have anxiety as a feature. In schizophrenia, for example, the patient may experience fear as a result of delusional thinking or hallucinations, or through insight into the illness with awareness of losses to self-esteem and autonomy. In a depressive disorder, anxiety is common with patients worrying over minor matters, and the anxiety may be linked to an inability to perform in work or social settings.

The incidence of substance abuse in the UK is high. Many patients first report symptoms of anxiety and mood disturbance and either do not reveal their use of alcohol or drugs or do not know their use of alcohol or drugs may be of significance. Sometimes patients may report that they have become dependent on alcohol or drugs as a way of controlling their anxiety.

COMMON FORMS OF ANXIETY

A broad distinction in the classification of anxiety disorders is made between anxiety which seems to be present most of the time and anxiety which only occurs in a particular place, or is tied to an actual event or anticipation of an event. OCD and post-traumatic stress disorder (PTSD) are also often grouped under the broad category of anxiety disorders (Table 2.3, overleaf).

Table 2.3. Anxiety disorders: a basic classification

Phobic disorders
Agoraphobia
- Unreasonably strong fear of specific places or events
- Patients often avoid these situations altogether
- Anxiety about being in places from which escape might be difficult or embarrassing
- Common fears – leaving home, crowds, travelling alone, open spaces

Social phobia
- Anxiety in social situations (small groups as opposed to crowds)
- Fear of inability to deal with the demands of the social situation
- May be specific difficulties, e.g. speaking or eating in public, or difficulties in all social situations

Specific phobia
- Anxiety restricted to specific situations, e.g. an object, procedure or situation
- Animals, heights, injections, flying

Generalized anxiety disorder
- Multiple symptoms of anxiety or tension
- Generalized 'free floating' anxiety
- Symptoms are often chronic and recur
- Often triggered by stressful events

Panic disorder
- Sudden attacks of severe anxiety, which begin suddenly and build rapidly
- Not situation specific
- Attacks last a few minutes associated with a need to leave the situation
- Avoidant behaviour may develop to prevent a further attack

OCD
- Persistent, distressing, intrusive thoughts, which the individual recognizes as their own; usually sees as irrational; tries to suppress or neutralize
- Repetitive behaviour or mental acts which the individual feels compelled to carry out; seen as irrational but temporarily reduces anxiety

Although the diagnoses set out in Table 2.3 have implications for both treatment and prognosis, the most common presentation of anxiety in primary care will be together with depressive symptoms. Treatment will often appropriately be that of the depressive disorder.

TREATMENT IN PRIMARY CARE

✓ Information and reassurance.
✓ Psychological interventions that can be done by the GP:
  – problem-solving,
  – slow breathing,
  – distraction,
  – simple exposure.
✓ Anxiolytic medication.
✓ Other interventions.

An important skill is the ability to listen carefully and with empathy. Feeling listened to and understood is particularly important for individuals with anxiety disorders who may feel inadequate, frightened and distressed. Once the GP has understood the nature of the problem and the patient's specific concerns, the management of anxiety disorders can be considered as a series of stages.

STAGE ONE: INFORMATION AND REASSURANCE

■ Appropriate explanation of symptoms.
■ Reassurance about the absence of physical illness.
■ Use of self-help leaflets to reinforce advice.

It is often helpful to have a well-rehearsed explanation of anxiety symptoms which is not complicated by an overly medical description. The following gives an example of what might be used:

Explaining anxiety

Anxiety can create a lot of symptoms which can worry us and make us think we are unwell. For instance, imagine if a man burst through the door brandishing a shot gun saying, 'That's it I've had enough of you two', we would both find our hearts missing a beat, we would find ourselves breathing faster, our hearts beating faster, we might get a lump in our throats, find it difficult to swallow, and we would begin to sweat ... This is a normal understandable reaction. We think we are in danger and our bodies' emergency system is switched on so we can run away or fight.

If I sat here when the man burst through the door and remained completely calm, you might think I was very brave. Knowing me I don't think this would be the right explanation ... I would only remain calm because I did not think the situation was dangerous, for instance, if I knew the man was an actor and this was the twentieth time he had burst in like this, rehearsing a GP-based soap opera.

This story tells us a number of things. The symptoms of anxiety are just like those of fear. The only difference with anxiety is that there is not an obvious cause. The story also points out how important our thoughts are in switching on the bodies' emergency system to cope with danger.

The most common causes for anxiety flaring up are: being over-loaded at work or home, relationship difficulties or having to face a worrying situation.

A GP should also explore with their patient, factors which may be important in understanding the onset and the maintenance of the anxiety disorder. Often this will involve asking about relationship difficulties, problems at home or difficulties at work. Beginning to talk can often on its own suggest changes, highlight problem-solving strategies or assist in coming to terms with problems or issues which will not change.

Education, advice and support have been shown to be as effective as anxiolytic medication for recent onset anxiety disorders (Catalan *et al.*, 1984). Similarly, GP treatment as usual (often just advice and support) has been shown to be as effective as both counselling (Friedli *et al.*, 1997) and problem-solving by practice nurses (Mynors-Wallis *et al.*, 1997) for recent-onset mixed anxiety and depressive disorders.

Self-help

- A stock of leaflets in the practice can be given to back up information given by the GP.
- Coping with panic (see advice below).
- A list of useful books for self-treatment of anxious symptoms is given at the end of the chapter. An ever-increasing amount of information is available over the internet.

For many patients the provision of appropriate information and reassurance may be a sufficient treatment in its own right, with a follow-up appointment to check all is well. For others, however, some psychological intervention and/or drug treatment may be necessary.

COPING WITH PANIC

When panic starts, sensible thinking stops! You cannot depend on being able to think clearly at this time. For this reason, you should read through the following rules very carefully *before* practising so that they are very clear in your mind. When you feel panicky, run through them again as slowly as you can. It can be a good idea to copy this list and to carry it around with you. If you have other ideas that you find are helpful, then add these to the list:

- *These feelings are normal bodily reactions.*
- They are not harmful.
- Don't add more frightening thoughts.
- Describe to yourself slowly what is happening.
- Wait for the fears to reduce, or even pass ... they will.
- Notice when the anxiety does actually fade.
- *Remember:* anxiety is unpleasant but not dangerous.

WHAT TO DO WHEN PANIC STARTS

- Remember that these feelings are nothing more than an exaggeration of the body's normal response to stress.
- These symptoms are not harmful or in the slightest way dangerous. They are very uncomfortable, but cannot do anything to you.
- Stop adding to your panic by thinking frightening thoughts, or by anticipating something awful is about to happen … it isn't!
- Try to slowly describe to yourself what is really happening in your body (not what you think is about to happen). Stick to the facts.
- Allow some time to pass without fighting it, or running away from it … try to accept it. Anxiety always comes to an end.
- Be aware that the anxiety is reducing. Remind yourself that you have coped with an unpleasant, but not dangerous, experience.

STAGE TWO: PSYCHOLOGICAL INTERVENTIONS THAT CAN BE DONE BY THE GP

- Simple problem-solving strategies.
- Advice about breathing.
- Distraction techniques and relaxation exercises.
- Simple exposure.

Simple problem-solving

Many patients develop anxiety in response to situational difficulties, and helping patients link symptoms to these difficulties may in itself begin to suggest changes. Problem-solving is described in more detail on page 31.

Advice about breathing

Hyperventilation may precipitate anxiety and is often a maintaining factor. Patients often describe the taking of deep breaths as a way of coping and then give a convincing demonstration of hyperventilation. Dizziness is a common symptom experienced by individuals who hyperventilate. Asking a patient to breathe quickly and shallowly for 30 seconds can often convincingly demonstrate the relationship between breathing and anxiety symptoms.

Patients should be given the following advice about slow breathing.

SLOW BREATHING TO REDUCE PHYSICAL SYMPTOMS OF ANXIETY

- Breathe in for 4 seconds and out for 4 seconds, pause for 4 seconds before breathing again.
- Practice 20 minutes morning and night (5–10 minutes is better than nothing).
- Use before and after situations that make you anxious.
- Regularly check and slow down breathing throughout the day.

Some patients also find it useful to cup their hands over mouth and nose as a way of regulating their breathing if they have begun to hyperventilate. The same can be achieved by using a paper bag; however, the use of cupped hands is less conspicuous.

Distraction

Worrying thoughts lead to anxious symptoms which in turn often worsen worrying thoughts. Distraction is a method which can be used to empty the mind of worrying thoughts and replace them with neutral thoughts.

DISTRACTION

Patients are asked to:
- Describe in detail to themselves a picture, a view or a story.
- Think of a relaxing image: the seashore, a lake or mountains.
- Save up worries for a circumscribed 'worry time' each day.

Relaxation can be thought of as a distraction technique. If the patient is focussing on tensing and relaxing muscles, or on a particular image, it is more difficult to be simultaneously worrying. There are a number of different techniques and a number of relaxation tapes available. Many local departments of clinical psychology will be able to provide copies of tapes, or recommend a commercially available tape. As with slow breathing, the patient should be encouraged to practice the relaxation techniques twice a day and implement them before and after anxiety provoking situations.

Simple exposure

Avoiding feared situations is an important factor in a large number of anxiety disorders. Each time a situation is avoided the idea is further strengthened in an individual's mind that they would have been overwhelmed by anxiety. Patients should be advised to face the feared situation and remain in it until either the anxiety subsides, or until they can convince themselves that they will not lose control or be unable to deal with the anxiety. Patients should be encouraged to repetitively place themselves in the feared situation.

The essential feature of exposure-based psychological treatments involves persuading the patient to stop avoiding the feared situation. Patients are told this will initially result in heightened levels of anxiety but will enable them to put 'to the test' predictions about losing control, going mad and so on. Repetitive exposure to the feared situation and a repetitive invalidation of feared consequences leads to a reduction in anticipatory anxiety, avoidance and disruption to an individual's life.

SIMPLE EXPOSURE

- Avoiding feared situations allows the fear to grow stronger.
- Confronting feared situations will reduce the fear.
- Draw up list of avoided situations.
- Start with easier tasks and build up to harder tasks.
- Face feared situation as often as possible.
- Remain in the situation.
- Experiencing anxiety allows prediction of 'loss of control' to be challenged.

Once patients have been given advice about exposure they can often take themselves through several tasks. In the initial stages, a friend or relative can often assist in the process; however, care should be taken that dependence does not develop or that being accompanied is not an avoidance.

CASE STUDY: LINDA

Linda was a 37-year-old woman who described herself as 'a bit of a worrier'. She was happily married, coping well with two boisterous under fives, and was working part time as a secretary. Four months ago she experienced a panic attack whilst at the supermarket. She left the trolley at the checkout , and went home fearing she was ill. She went to casualty later the same day, was discharged after some basic tests, and told it was probably 'due to stress'. Since then she had experienced two further panic attacks and had begun to avoid, not only going to supermarkets, but also going out alone.

Dr Smith listened to her story. He checked for the presence of depressive symptoms. In that Linda's symptoms were largely anxiety, he then provided an explanation of panic attacks. This was backed up by a leaflet. Linda was reassured that she was not going mad, and that she did not have a serious physical illness.

At a second appontment, Linda felt sufficient trust in Dr Smith to embark on a simple exposure based-programme which included daily targets about going out. Initially, a friend accompanied her to the corner shop, then to larger shops further away from home and then she went alone. Dr Smith outlined how important it was for her to get anxious in these situations as this was the only way she could prove to herself that all of the things she dreaded happening would not actually occur.

After 1 week Linda came back to the surgery feeling very pleased with her progress. She had been reassured and felt that she had been understood. She had placed herself in a number of situations which she would have previously avoided, and whilst she had got anxious and panicky, she began to believe she would not be overwhelmed by the symptoms, and had begun to feel a sense of mastery over her life once more. A further appointment was spent going over some of the same material about anxiety and setting more challenging tasks built upon the initial progress.

Lessons from the case study
- Check for depressive symptoms in anxiety.
- Education and advice are helpful.
- Simple behavioural treatment involving exposure with response prevention is possible in primary care without specialist referral.

STAGE THREE: ANXIOLYTIC MEDICATION

If simple psychological interventions are ineffective, or if the patient is too anxious to use the techniques, medication may be used.

- Antidepressant drugs.
- Benzodiazepines.
- Betablockers.
- Neuroleptics.
- Buspirone.

All drugs used for the treatment of anxiety have a strong placebo effect, hence patients may benefit from drugs despite little evidence for a specific anxiolytic action.

Antidepressant drugs

Anxious and depressive symptoms go hand in hand in primary care. It is unsurprising, therefore, that drugs effective in the treatment of depression are also effective in the treatment of anxiety. Some of the antidepressant drugs have a specific indication for anxiety, but there is no evidence that these drugs are more effective than other antidepressants not specifically licensed for this purpose. Antidepressant drugs with a sedative effect, e.g. amitriptyline or trazodone, may be helpful if sleep is a problem, or if some initial daytime sedation is needed.

On introduction, some antidepressants can cause an initial worsening of anxiety and panic. A useful rule of thumb is to start at a low dose (half the therapeutic dose in the case of SSRIs) or, for example, 10 mg or 25 mg of amitriptyline. The final dose that is required may be the full therapeutic dose, or even higher, but tolerance will be better if low doses are used in the first instance.

Antidepressants for anxiety may take longer to take effect than for the treatment of a depressive disorder. A pragmatic guide to prescribing is given below.

ANTIDEPRESSANTS FOR ANXIETY

- Try a TCA: imipramine or amitriptyline, first line.
- Start at the low dose of 25 mg day but increase by 25 mg every 3 or 4 days depending on the response and side-effects.
- If a TCA is contraindicated or not tolerated, start an SSRI at half the usual therapeutic dose, and increase to the therapeutic dose after 1 week as necessary.
- Wait for 6–8 weeks at the maximum tolerated dose (within BNF limits) before concluding the drug is ineffective.

Benzodiazepines

Benzodiazepines are effective anxiolytics; however, the risks of tolerance and dependence are now well known. Benzodiazepines should only be used for the short-term relief of severe anxiety.

Betablockers

Although there is little formal evidence for the use of betablockers for the treatment of anxiety, propranolol at a dose of 20–60 mg is widely used. Doses above 80 mg a day may lead to respiratory and cardiac symptoms. Some patients may experience vivid dreams. Betablockers are most effective for patients with autonomic complaints, particularly tachycardia.

Neuroleptics

Low-dose neuroleptics have been widely used as anxiolytics. Even in low doses, however, neuroleptics may cause tardive dyskinesia and there are risks of cardiotoxicity. Hence neuroleptics should be used cautiously, if at all, in the treatment of anxiety.

Buspirone

Buspirone is a 5-HT agonist. It has a slow onset of action and may take 4 weeks at 30 mg per day to start working optimally. It may have a role in the treatment of chronic generalized anxiety disorder.

STAGE FOUR: OTHER INTERVENTIONS

If simple psychological and drug interventions are ineffective or not fully effective, local community or primary care-based resources may help, these will depend on locally available resources.

POSSIBLE PRIMARY CARE RESOURCES

- Relaxation classes.
- Stress management groups.
- Self-help groups.
- Activity programmes at leisure centres.
- Yoga.

Despite its widespread use, there is little evidence that applied relaxation (a technique involving the imagination of relaxing situations to induce muscular and mental relaxation) is of clinical benefit. The value of applied relaxation may stem from placebo and non-specific effects.

OBSESSIVE COMPULSIVE DISORDER (OCD)

The essential features of OCD are recurrent, persistent and intrusive thoughts and/or repetitive behaviours. The patient for at least some of the time sees these thoughts and/or behaviours as excessive or unreasonable. The patient often tries to suppress or resist the thoughts and behaviours but finds that this leads to heightened levels of anxiety. Some patients may not tell anyone about their symptoms fearing it is a sign of madness.

However, others, especially those with exaggerated thoughts of possible illness, may repetitively seek reassurance from their GP and others.

OCD

- May be secondary to a depressive disorder.
- Most need to be referred to clinical psychologists or CMHTs.
- Consider clomipramine or SSRIs.
- A significant number of patients will have a chronic course, and numerous 'failures to engage in therapy'.

OCD can be an extremely severe and limiting condition; however, less severe cases may take on a fluctuating course without any intervention. With the vast majority of cases, help should be sought through a CMHT. The most successful interventions are psychological, most commonly involving behavioural and cognitive behavioural therapies.

5-HT reuptake blockers, either clomipramine or SSRIs (fluvoxamine, fluoxetine, paroxetine and sertraline), have a beneficial effect on symptoms of OCD. Patients may need a minimum of 12 weeks on these antidepressants, and on higher doses than in the treatment of depression for there to be any evidence of benefit. There is no evidence for or against the use of combined psychological and drug treatments.

In very rare cases of the most severe OCD, psycho-surgical interventions have been used.

POST-TRAUMATIC STRESS DISORDER (PTSD)

After any trauma it is normal to experience a number of emotions and symptoms including marked anxiety, feelings of numbness and detachment, not wanting to think about the trauma and experiencing intrusive, vivid recollections of the traumatic event. With most people these symptoms diminish over a few weeks. However, for some people a number of these symptoms persist over time. Symptoms are categorized under three headings:

- Re-experiencing of the traumatic event.
- Avoidance of stimuli associated with the event and a general numbing of responsiveness.
- Increased arousal.

PTSD

- Precipitant is a life-threatening trauma.
- Re-experiencing symptoms: flashbacks, nightmares, intrusive thoughts.
- Avoidance symptoms: numbness, detachment, physical avoidance of situations.
- Increased arousal symptoms: irritability, sleep disturbance, hypervigilance, startle response.
- Symptom duration at least 1 month.

There are no clear indicators to predict who will be likely to experience PTSD and it is important to remember that there may be an interval of apparently normal functioning between the trauma and the symptoms developing. It is also important that a possible neurological cause is excluded if there has been any type of head injury.

When a patient experiences a traumatic event a listening and empathic approach, in addition to practical help, may be all that is required. If there is evidence to suggest PTSD, onward referral to a clinical psychologist or therapist with special knowledge of the treatment of PTSD should be arranged. If trauma is a result of work or accident, private referral may be possible.

Most psychological forms of treatment involve encouraging the individual to recall and/or re-experience the trauma repetitively and to 'emotionally process' traumatic material. A number of organizations offer psychological debriefing hoping to decrease the risk of individuals developing PTSD in the few days following a trauma, e.g. staff held up in a robbery in a bank, or ambulance staff who attended a major disaster. There is no evidence to support such interventions, and they may make symptoms worse.

Whilst most people do recover from PTSD, there are a small number of people who continue to experience their symptoms chronically for many years.

REFERRING PATIENTS TO SPECIALIST SERVICES

For patients who do not respond to treatment in primary care, or patients whose anxiety is severe, intractable or for whom background factors seem complex, onward referral should be considered to more specialist care. It may be possible to refer patients directly to clinical psychologists or to individuals within a CMHT.

WHO TO REFER

- Patients with OCD and PTSD.
- Patients with severe, persisting symptoms.

A frustration for many GPs is the difficulty they have accessing help for patients with severe anxiety disorders. Many specialist teams in the UK only take on for treatment those patients considered to be seriously mentally ill and there can often be long waiting lists for appointments with clinical psychologists.

A large number of GP practices in the UK now have in-house counselling services, and some research suggests there may be benefits from counselling for patients with anxiety which may be maintained over time (Baker et al., 1998). Randomized controlled trials suggest, however, little additional benefit for counselling over and above treatment as usual by the GP (Friedli et al., 1997), although evidence is increasing that patients with depressive disorders may benefit from counselling (see page 34).

REFERENCES

Baker R, Allen H, Gibson S *et al.*, (1998). Evaluation of a primary care counselling service in Dorset. *British Journal of General Practice* **48**:1049–54.

Catalan J, Gath D, Edmonds G, Ennis J (1984). The effect of non-prescribing of anxiolytics in general practice. *British Journal of Psychiatry* **144**:593–602.

Friedli K, King M, Lloyd M *et al.*, (1997). Randomised controlled assessment of non-directive psychotherapy versus routine GP care. *Lancet* **350**:1662–5.

Lloyd KR, Jenkins R, Mann A (1996). Long term outcome of patients with neurotic illness in general practice. *British Medical Journal* **313**:26–8.

Meltzer H, Gill B, Petticrew M (1995). *OPCS surveys of psychiatric morbidity in Great Britain report. No 1. The prevalence of psychiatric morbidity amongst adults aged 16 to 64 living in private households in Great Britain.* HMSO, London.

Mynors-Wallis LM, Gath D, Davies I, Gray A, Barbour F (1997). A randomised controlled trial and cost analysis of problem-solving treatment given by community nurses for emotional disorders in primary care. *British Journal of Psychiatry* **170**:113–19.

FURTHER READING

Anon (1997). Stopping Panic Attacks. *Drugs and Therapeutics Bulletin* **35**:58–61.

Baker R (1995), *Understanding Panic Attacks and Overcoming Fear.* Lion Publishing, Oxford.

Breton S (1986). *Don't Panic: a Guide to Overcoming Panic Attacks.* McDonald and Co, London.

Butler G, Hope A (1995). *Manage Your Mind.* OUP, Oxford.

Marks I (1995). *Living with Fear.* McGraw Hill, Maidenhead.

Priest R (1996). *Anxiety and Depression.* McDonald and Co, London.

Weekes C (1995). *Self-Help for your Nerves.* Angus and Robertson.

WEBSITES

Royal College of Psychiatrists
www.rcpsych.ac.uk/public/help/anxiety/anxiety.htm
Useful information on a range of mental disorders.

Anxiety Disorders Association of America
www.adaa.org
Self-help and information site.

OCD Resource Centre
www.ocdresource.com
Gives information about OCD.

SELF-HELP

The Anxiety Disorders Association (ANXIA)
20 Church Street, Dagenham, Essex RM10 9UR
Tel: 020 8491 4700 (enquiries)
    020 8270 0999 (helpline)

First Steps to Freedom
22 Randall Road, Kenilworth, Warwickshire CV8 1JY
Tel: 01926 864473 (administration)
    01926 851608 (helpline)
Website: www.firststeps.demon.co.uk
Offers self-help to sufferers from anxiety disorders.

National Phobics Society
4 Cheltenham Road, Chorlton, Manchester M21 9QN
Tel: 0161 881 1937
Website: www.phobics-society.org.uk

No Panic (Local Groups)
93 Brands Farm Way, Randlay, Telford, Shropshire TF3 3JQ
Tel: 01952 590005
    01952 590545 (helpline)
Helpline, information booklets and local self-help groups for people with anxiety phobias, obsessions and panic.

chapter 3

The psychotic patient

- The importance of early recognition.
- Use of the Mental Health Act.
- Role of primary care in the management of patients with a chronic psychotic illness.
- Risk assessment .
- Appropriate use of new antipsychotic drugs.

INTRODUCTION

Psychotic symptoms are found in several psychiatric diagnoses: schizophrenia, delusional disorder, drug-induced psychosis, affective disorders (mania and depression) and dementia. Usually, specialist services are involved in attempting to make broad diagnostic sense of psychotic symptoms. The GP, however, has a key role to play in detecting psychotic symptoms, arranging appropriate referral, and in the continuing management of patients with chronic psychotic disorders. Details about the specific management of depressive and manic disorders, dementia and substance misuse will be found in the relevant chapters.

Epidemiology

Table 3.1. Epidemiology of schizophrenia

Lifetime risk: just under 1 in 100

Peak onset age: 15–45 years (earlier in men)

Risk factors: family history, obstetric complications

Number of patients on the average GP's list: 8 (prevalence is much higher in urban areas)

Risk of suicide: x9 population mean (12% of all deaths)

Despite the emphasis in UK community care on patients with severe mental illness, approximately one-third of patients with schizophrenia are no longer in contact with secondary services.

Recognition and diagnosis

✓ Early recognition.
✓ Acute psychotic disorders.
✓ Chronic psychotic disorders.
✓ Diagnostic criteria of schizophrenia.

Early recognition of psychotic symptoms

The first presentation of a psychotic illness is an unusual event in primary care. The average GP will see a new case of psychosis once every 4–5 years.

There is now increasing evidence that if psychotic symptoms are detected at an early stage and treated appropriately, the long-term outcome for the disorder will be improved (Birchwood *et al.*, 1997). The

GP is clearly a key to such early recognition. The first symptoms of a developing psychotic illness may well not be frank delusions or hallucinations, but rather an insidious deterioration in social functioning. Patients may become increasingly withdrawn, apathetic, lose contact with friends or be unable to cope with work. Patients with a developing early psychotic illness rarely self-present and often only come to the attention of the GP through the concerns of family and friends. Occasionally, the patient may present with an odd or bizarre physical problem.

Sometimes psychotic symptoms are obvious either from speaking to relatives or from the patient themselves. However, patients, particularly in the early stages of their illness, often can make little sense of their experiences. The use of open questions is important in eliciting symptoms, e.g.:

'Is there anything particular troubling you?'
'Are you feeling concerned about anything?'
'Are you frightened or anxious about anything?'
'Do you feel people are out to harm you in any way, or to get at you?'
'Are you having any unusual experiences that you cannot explain?'

In the absence of clear psychotic symptoms patients may be troubled by a sense of unease, a feeling that something is about to happen. This is delusional mood, which may precede the formation of clear delusional beliefs.

EARLY RECOGNITION OF PSYCHOTIC SYMPTOMS

- Deterioration in social functioning.
- Help seeking by relatives.
- Abnormal mental state: perceptual abnormalities, ideas of reference, delusional mood.
- Odd personality.

The GP may simply have a gut feeling that something is not right or the patient seems odd. This may well merit at least a telephone call for discussion and advice from specialist services.

The acute onset of frank psychotic symptoms often results in requests for an emergency assessment. Alternatively, patients may be picked up by the police and assessed by police surgeons. All such patients should be assessed by specialist services.

DIAGNOSIS

The primary care version of ICD-10 makes the simple diagnostic distinction between acute and chronic psychotic disorders.

ACUTE PSYCHOTIC DISORDER

Recent onset of:
- Hallucinations.
- Delusions.
- Agitation or bizarre behaviour.
- Disorganized or strange speech.
- Extreme and labile emotional states.

Presenting complaints may be from:
- Patients: hearing voices, strange beliefs, confusion, apprehension.
- Families: strange behaviour, withdrawal, suspiciousness, threats.

CHRONIC PSYCHOTIC DISORDER

Chronic problems:
- Social withdrawal.
- Low motivation or interest.
- Self-neglect.
- Disordered thinking.

Periodic episodes of:
- Agitation or restlessness.
- Bizarre behaviour.
- Hallucinations.
- Delusions.

Presenting complaints may be from:
- Patients: difficulty with thinking or concentration, hearing voices, strange beliefs, problems with medication.
- Families: apathy, withdrawal, poor hygiene, strange behaviour.

The specific diagnosis of schizophrenia is a difficult one to make and often all the diagnostic criteria only become apparent after a fairly lengthy and detailed assessment. This will almost always involve specialist services. The broad outline of the diagnostic criteria for schizophrenia is given in Table 3.2.

Table 3.2. Diagnostic criteria of schizophrenia

Symptoms
- Positive: hallucinations, delusions, two present for at least 1 month
- Negative: poor self-care, social withdrawal, poor motivation, blunting of affect
- Disorganization: behaviour, speech

Social dysfunction

Duration
- ICD-10: active symptoms for at least 1 month
- DSM-IV: active symptoms for at least 6 months

Exclude other diagnoses
Affective, organic, etc.

Other specific diagnoses to consider in the psychotic patient are manic and depressive psychotic disorders in which there are prominent affective symptoms, delusional disorders and drug-induced psychoses.

Delusional disorders, which used to be known as paranoid disorders, comprise a separate diagnostic group. The symptoms are of a persisting delusional belief in the absence of any perceptual abnormalities. The delusional beliefs are often circumscribed and patients may continue to lead relatively normal lives.

Drug induced psychoses. Many illicit drugs (particularly stimulants) cause psychotic symptoms. Patients with psychotic symptoms need to be safely managed whatever the supposed aetiology. Hence a specialist referral is still indicated even if a drug aetiology is suspected.

MANAGEMENT IN PRIMARY CARE

Patients with psychotic disorders can be considered in three groups with regards to their management in primary care.

Approximately one-third have a single psychotic episode which is acute in onset, short lived and often precipitated by a stressful life event. Such episodes respond well to treatment. Patients should be advised that they may have an increased susceptibility to develop a psychotic episode in response to the use of illicit drugs.

A second group will have a chronic but well-controlled psychotic disorder. These will be patients who are on long-term antipsychotic medication. Such patients may be in contact with a practice nurse, administering depot medication. These patients may not be in regular contact with secondary care, but may need to be referred for advice regarding medication and side-effects.

A third group are those with a chronic psychotic disorder who show only a partial or incomplete response to treatment. The needs of this group are often complex and cover both health and social care. Patients within this group should have ongoing support from secondary services.

Acute psychotic symptoms should be referred to specialist services for diagnosis, risk assessment and advice about appropriate treatments. The GP needs to ensure that the patient and carers are safe – ask for an urgent assessment under the Mental Health Act if necessary. Whilst awaiting advice and support from the specialist services, attempt to minimize stress and confrontation. Consider antipsychotic or antianxiety medication to relieve symptoms and agitation.

Patients with chronic psychotic disorders, will inevitably be managed, at least in part, in primary care. Burns and Kendrick (1997) have set out a gold standard guideline for the care of chronic schizophrenia in general practice.

GUIDELINES FOR THE CARE OF CHRONIC SCHIZOPHRENIA

- Identifying your patients and organizing a regular review.
- Comprehensive assessment:
  - physical problems,
  - mental state,
  - social factors,
  - medication.
- Information and advice for patients and carers.
- Indications for involving specialist services.
- Crisis management.

Identifying your patients and organizing a regular review

It has been shown that about 90% of identifiable patients with long-term mental illness can be found by:

- Asking the primary care team who has been suffering a long-time from a major psychiatric illness.
- A review of the repeat prescriptions for antipsychotic medication.
- Using a diagnostic register if it exists.

Such a list could form the basis of a discussion within the primary care team and the CMHT as to who is involved with such patients and the arrangment of an appropriate plan of care. It is yet to be established that calling such patients in for regular 6 monthly or annual reviews is of benefit.

Comprehensive assessment

The purpose of such an assessment is not that the GP should take over the role of the specialist services, but that problems should be identified that can be brought to the attention of whoever is best placed to support the patient.

Physical problems – including alcohol and drugs

Patients with schizophrenia have an unhealthy lifestyle (Brown *et al.*, 1999) with an increased rate of mortality from natural causes due to cigarette and alcohol use, lack of exercise and poor diet.

Advising about and treating these lifestyle and physical problems may be the most useful intervention in primary care. Patients with schizophrenia may need a proactive and targeted approach.

PHYSICAL CARE FOR PATIENTS WITH CHRONIC PSYCHOTIC DISORDER

- Health promotion: cigarettes, alcohol.
- Obesity: exercise, diet, nutrition.
- Cardiovascular: hypertension.
- Teeth and feet.

Mental state

Specific enquiry should be made about positive symptoms present, e.g. 'Do your beliefs about … continue to trouble you?', or 'Are the voices still a problem? Getting worse?' Identification of low mood and suicidal thoughts is important – patients with schizophrenia have a mortality risk of suicide nine times that of the general population. An assessment of self-neglect, apathy and withdrawal should be made.

Social and environmental factors

There are several factors to consider including accommodation, daily activities, housing and benefits advice.

Review of medication, adherence and side-effects

Table 3.3. Antipsychotic medication

Traditional antipsychotic drugs
Chlorpromazine
Trifluoperazine
Haloperidol

Side-effects
- Extrapyramidal: acute dystonia, akathisia, parkinsonian syndrome, tardive dyskinesia
- Anticholinergic
- Antiadrenergic
- Sedative

Advantages: long history of established efficacy with positive symptoms, cheap
Disadvantages: side-effects, not good for negative symptoms

Sulpiride
Sulpiride is less likely to cause extrapyramidal side-effects, and is less sedative and anticholinergic than the traditional antipsychotics. The evidence for its efficacy is less well established than that for many other antipsychotics

Depot neuroleptics
Flupenthixol decanoate (Depixol)
Fluphenazine decanoate (Modecate)
Haloperidol decanoate (Haldol)
Zuclopenthixol decanoate (Clopixol)

The advantage of depot administration is known compliance, with an associated reduction in relapse and readmission rates. The disadvantages include stigma and the lack of quick reductions in dose if side-effects develop

Continued on page 80

Table 3.3 (*continued*)

Atypical neuroleptics

Risperidone	Quetiapine
Olanzapine	Amisulpride

The term 'atypical' refers to a group of neuroleptic drugs with less extrapyramidal side-effects than the traditional neuroleptics, with no reduction in efficacy. The drugs may be more effective at treating negative symptoms. The improved tolerability may result in improved adherence and hence a reduction in relapse and readmission

Clozapine

An atypical neuroleptic with proven effectiveness in treatment-resistant schizophrenia. It can cause a, usually reversible, neutropenia in 3% of patients which may lead to agranulocytosis. It can only be prescribed within the framework of the Clozaril Patient Monitoring Service, with weekly haematological monitoring for 18 weeks, fortnightly monitoring to a year and 4-weekly monitoring thereafter if all is well. Other side-effects include sedation and seizures

Information and advice for patients and carers

Patients and carers should be given information about local voluntary organizations, such as MIND, NSF and SANE. Parents need to be assured that they are not to blame. Carers may need advice about the negative aspects of schizophrenia which are often perceived as laziness and hence more difficult to cope with than more florid positive symptoms. Patients and their carers may also need help, advice and information regarding accessing welfare and benefits. In the UK, the National Service Framework for Mental Health states that all carers should receive an annual carer's assessment and have their own care plan to meet any identified needs.

Indications for involving specialist services
See 'When to refer' (page 83).

Crisis management

Planning for a crisis

- Ensure clear mechanisms are in place for obtaining specialist help in an emergency (agreed with secondary care services and written down):
  - identify day and night contact numbers for mental health services and social services,
  - consider the status and experience of the secondary care professional who will review the patient,
  - consider whether the review takes place in the home, casualty department, or hospital ward – is there a risk of violence?
- Ensure the carers know who to contact.
- Carry oral and parenteral tranquillizers and anticholinergics, and Mental Health Act forms in the night bag.

Acute situation

- Assess the risk of self-harm or violence before seeing the patient:
  - check the medical records for previous episodes,
  - discuss the situation with carers and other professionals.
- Ensure physical help is available if needed (ask for the police to accompany you if concerned).
- Avoid being left with the patient with no quick exit route.
- Assess whether the patient's mental state has changed or not.
- Consider drug treatment if the patient is willing.
- Consider informal admission.
- If compulsory admission indicated:
  - contact the duty approved social worker,
  - contact the duty consultant psychiatrist or other section 12 approved doctor.

Review the crisis and identify any lessons to be learnt for future crises.

USE OF THE MENTAL HEALTH ACT (SEE APPENDIX)

- The Mental Health Act can be used for an assessment, e.g. if you are not sure what is happening, the patient is refusing to see you and the relatives are concerned.
- The Mental Health Act can be implemented on the grounds of risk to health alone, it is *not* necessary for there to be a risk to self or others.
- The patient's relatives can request an assessment under the Mental Health Act by contacting their local social services department.

ROLE OF PRACTICE NURSE

In some practices, the practice nurse will administer depot medication (in other services this is a role undertaken by community mental health nurses). It is important if the practice nurse does administer the depot that she is trained to assess the patient's mental and physical health as well as to monitor drug side-effects. There should be a clear protocol for action in case of poor compliance or other concerns.

DRIVING AND PSYCHOTIC ILLNESS

In the UK, the Driver and Vehicle Licensing Agency (DVLA) must be notified following an acute psychotic episode. The patient's driving licence may be withdrawn until the patient has been well for up to 12 months. In chronic schizophrenia, driving is usually permitted provided that the patient is compliant with medication, their condition is stable and symptoms do not affect driving ability. It is the patient who has the duty to inform the DVLA, but the doctor may be sufficiently concerned to contact the DVLA directly. A breach in patient confidentiality is weighed up against public safety.

WHEN TO REFER

- Relapse:
  - a 'relapse signature' may have been identified by the patient. These will be the early signs of an impending relapse, e.g. sleeping poorly, a sense of unease,
  - sudden or gradual changes in behaviour.
- Increased risk of relapse:
  - poor adherence to treatment,
  - major life events,
  - family conflict.
- Review of medication:
  - persistent symptoms,
  - persistent side-effects,
  - poly-pharmacy,
  - 5-yearly consultant reviews.
- Concurrent substance or alcohol misuse.
- Newly registered patients with psychotic illness.
- Any problem the GP cannot deal with.

WHAT TO EXPECT FROM SECONDARY CARE

- ✓ CPA.
- ✓ Risk assessment.
- ✓ Shared care.
- ✓ Shared prescribing.

Patients with schizophrenia and chronic psychotic illnesses form a large part of the workload of specialist mental health services. Specialist services should ensure such patients are a priority for receiving their services.

The following should be available in all areas:

- Prompt assessment of new referrals and of known patients identified as being of concern.
- Assessment to include diagnosis, social factors and risk, leading to an appropriate management plan.
- Ongoing involvement for all patients in the early stage of their illness ensuring co-ordination of appropriate services.
- Ongoing involvement for all patients with a history of:
  - risk to selves or others,
  - concurrent substance misuse,
  - poor adherence to treatment plans,
  - poor social network/support.
- Shared care of patients in a stable phase of their illness with easy access to specialist advice for:
  - medication,
  - psychological treatment for patient and carers,
  - daytime activities,
  - welfare benefits.
- Assessment and support for carers.
- The management of all patients under the care of specialist services in England is within the framework of the Care Programme Approach (CPA).

CPA

All patients in contact with specialist mental health services should receive:

- An assessment of health and social needs.
- A care plan to meet such needs.
- A care co-ordinator to ensure the care plan is implemented.
- Regular review of the plan.

There are two levels of CPA: standard CPA for patients with

straight-forward care plans and enhanced CPA for those patients with complex needs. The care plan should include action to be taken in a crisis and advice to the GP as to how to access additional help.

RISK AND RISK ASSESSMENT IN SCHIZOPHRENIA

A contemporary theme running through all health services at present is risk assessment and management. The Christopher Clunis case particularly highlighted this issue for community mental health services following the murder of Jonathan Zito. This tragedy and similar events have been widely reported and cited as a failure of community care by the media. Unfortunately, certain sections of the general public now believe that the term schizophrenia is synonymous with murderous intent. Such a perception is far from the true position as established in a report by Taylor and Gunn (1999) which found that the homicide rate by persons with serious mental illness has remained relatively stable for the past 35 years. Mental illness accounts for a tiny part (about 3%) of the factors predicting violence. To protect the public it would be much better to lock up young men rather than patients with schizophrenia.

It is part of the remit of specialist services to assess and establish risk in all patients referred, and undertake on-going risk assessments for patients in their care.

An assessment of risk will generally concentrate on three main areas:

- The risk of self-harm.
- The risk that the patient might pose towards other people, i.e. their partner, children, carer, relatives, persons that the patient has delusional ideas about and, lastly, random members of the public.
- The risk of self-neglect perhaps through depression or the negative symptoms of their illness.

The assessment of risk should lead to a management plan to moderate and minimize the risk. Factors that increase or decrease risk are not all illness related, and may relate to the patient's social situation, relationships, coping ability, substance misuse and pre-morbid personality.

RISK FACTORS FOR VIOLENCE TO OTHERS

- Certain psychotic symptoms, e.g. command hallucinations, persecutory delusions.
- Previous history of violence.
- History of threats.
- Escalating conflict with specific individuals, e.g. vulnerable carer.
- Alcohol and drug use.
- Poor adherence with care plans.

RISK FACTORS FOR SUICIDE

- Suicidal ideas and plans.
- Early in illness.
- Recent hospital discharge.
- Poor adherence with care plan.
- Past history of suicide attempts.
- Recent stress-related life events or losses.
- Alcohol and drug use.

SHARED CARE

How to involve specialist services

If the patient will not see a psychiatrist, they might be persuaded to see a community mental health nurse either in the surgery or at home. A preliminary discussion between the GP and a member of the CMHT may indicate the best way of setting up the initial engagement.

The importance of the initial assessment cannot be overstated when dealing with someone who may be developing a psychotic illness. The assessment need not be completed on the first consultation – it can be continued over several meetings. It is a relatively simple task to be able to see that someone is unwell, but it is not necessarily easy to engage, assess and take a history.

The case history below is written by a psychiatric nurse who works in the community and is attached to a GP practice. The case study illustrates that that an experienced nurse with time and commitment is able to gain the trust of the patient, an understanding of the family and is able to establish the level of risk.

CASE STUDY: SARAH

Sarah was first seen at a regular psychiatric liaison clinic in the health centre at the request of her GP. He thought that something was not quite right, adding that she was an odd girl from an odd family. Sarah was a tall, 23-year-old, unemployed, single woman who lived with her mother, aunt and uncle. She was casually dressed, slightly over-weight and had the appearance of the early stages of neglect. Sarah said that she had finally decided to come to see me because she was having problems going out on her own, particularly after dark.

Sarah's father had deserted her mother before she was born and they had never met. Sarah said that she had not enjoyed school very much as she was bullied. In her teenage years she had started to truant and had left school at 15. Sarah worked for a short while in a florists and then in a hotel kitchen. She found this work to be very stressful and gave up the job after 7 weeks. She had not been in paid employment since. Sarah attended a day centre run by the local MIND group which provided her with somewhere to go, a cheap, substantial meal and free access to a pool table. During her attendance at the day centre, Sarah developed some negative views about mental health services having heard many of the members tell of their experiences.

Sarah was clear that she wanted help with her anxiety, but was not initially able to state what was making her anxious. She did say that several months previously some youths on motorcycles had gathered outside her house, late one night and had made a lot of noise revving their bike engines. Sarah went to speak to them about the noise and was knocked to the ground and kicked. Since that incident, Sarah had taken to carrying a stiletto flick knife in her handbag for her protection.

In an unguarded moment Sarah said that there was an alien presence around her house, and immediately seemed embarrassed and upset and said that she could not say any more. In an agitated state she then got up to leave saying, 'You can't make me take medication you know, you can only do that on section.' I asked Sarah if I could see her again. Sarah said that there was no way she was coming to the hospital but I said that I could see her at home.

The home visit to Sarah took place a week later. Sarah's house, in a well-kept suburb, was in contrast to the others in the street. The garden was overgrown and badly faded paint was peeling from the front door and window frames. Sarah reported being anxious as a result of the many strange beliefs that she held and said she was unable to talk to people about these beliefs because of a fear of being ridiculed. Sarah was concerned that the disclosure of any of her beliefs would lead to her being put on a section of the Mental Health Act. Sarah had noticed that her patterns of thought had changed and thought that this might have been due to additives that were in processed food. As a result of this belief, it took Sarah a great deal of time to do her grocery shopping as every item she bought had to be examined to see if it contained any of the substances which she believed had affected her mental functioning. At particularly bad times, Sarah said that her diet had been quite restricted. Sarah also described being unable to use the bath in her house as she thought that the water supply had been contaminated during recent maintenance work – the water supply had been cut off for a few hours and when the supply was restored it was initially discoloured.

Sarah's mother joined the assessment unannounced. 'What rubbish has she been telling you, she needs a job not happy pills?' was the mother's opening statement. In the presence of her mother Sarah seemed to be apprehensive and ill at ease. After a few minutes and a discussion with her mother, I asked Sarah if we could meet again and she agreed, saying that she felt a little better for having spoken to someone.

During the next few weeks, I was a frequent visitor to Sarah's home. It became evident that Sarah was the butt of a lot of criticism within the house and that at times her uncle was openly hostile towards her. Sarah's mental state fluctuated, but when her mood began to drop I worried that she might harm herself or others. Sarah's self-care deteriorated and she stopped going out. She was still reluctant to consider any form of medical treatment. Sarah stopped washing and developed a fungal infection in her groin. She finally agreed to a hospital admission providing we treated her physical ailments.

Sarah initially settled on the ward but within 48 hours she wanted to leave saying that she was going to the multi-storey car park and throw herself over the top. The response to this was to detain Sarah under section of the Mental Health Act. She was then treated with antipsychotic medication and made a slow but sustained recovery. Eventually she agreed to be discharged to sheltered accommodation, where she continues to live taking her medication and supported by the CMHT.

Lessons from the case study
- Early recognition – 'odd girl'.
- Early engagement and development of trust by the patient.
- Increased understanding of the role of the family.
- Ongoing and changing risk assessment.
- Use of hospital and the Mental Health Act.

Clinics in primary care

GPs and psychiatrists often value clinics held in the surgery rather than in the outpatient department. Psychologists and mental health nurses also have shifted clinics into primary care.

Holding a regular clinic in primary care reduces the stigma surrounding the mental health services. It also improves integration and communication between primary and secondary care. Most importantly, it reduces non-attendance because access to community mental health care is as easy as going to the doctor. A further benefit is that such a service development promotes earlier effective interventions.

The model of specialist clinics in primary care can be adapted to local needs, ranging from simply a shifted outpatient clinic to a much closer liaison role.

Shared prescribing

The psychiatrist should be aware of the antipsychotic drugs available, and their advantages and side-effects. It is often the case that GPs continue to prescribe drugs started in specialist care. If this occurs it is important that:

- Drug doses are kept under regular review:
  - the need to continue,
  - dose adjustment,
  - the management of side-effects.
- Agreement is reached about the appropriate prescribing of the new atypical drugs. The shared care guidelines agreed in Dorset between psychiatrists and GPs on the appropriate prescribing of atypical antipsychotics are given in Figure 3.1. The guidelines attempt to set out good practice, whilst recognizing the cost implications of unlimited prescribing of these drugs.

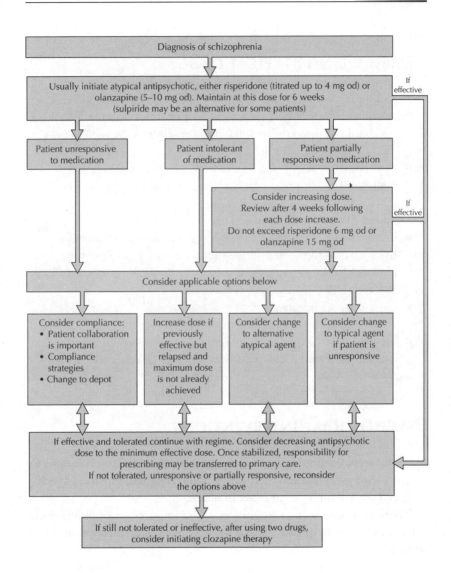

Figure 3.1. Drug treatment of newly diagnosed schizophrenia.

Prescribing atypical drugs

Atypical antipsychotics are relatively expensive but should have a clear and agreed role in the management of schizophrenia. The drugs should be used in the following situations:

- First episode schizophrenia: although the evidence is not yet available it is important that patients with a new diagnosis of schizophrenia should be given drugs they can tolerate. It is hoped that this will improve long-term compliance.
- Troublesome extra-pyramidal side-effects on typical neuroleptics: a trial of sulpiride may be indicated which has fewer extra-pyramidal side-effects than many of the older drugs, but may also be a less-effective antipsychotic.
- Unresponsive negative symptoms: the atypical drugs may be somewhat better at reducing negative symptoms
- Treatment refractory schizophrenia: clozapine should be considered if two antipsychotic drugs have failed.

Psychosocial interventions

Specialist services should provide a range of psychosocial interventions for patients with psychosis and their carers. Some areas will provide a specific, targetted service for a recent onset of illness.

There is an increasing recognition of the importance of psychosocial interventions for both patients and their families. Such interventions may include:

- Education programmes: for patients and carers.
- Family interventions:
  - supporting carers,
  - reducing criticism of patients (decreasing over-involvement and expressed emotion),
  - practical support.

- Cognitive behavioural therapy for patients with persistent symptoms. This will attempt to provide:
  - enhanced coping skills,
  - realistic goal setting,
  - a rationale for symptoms,
  - the modification of delusional beliefs.
- Compliance therapy: specific interventions to improve adherence to medication.

REFERENCES

Birchwood M, McGorry P, Jackson H (1997). Early intervention in schizophrenia. *British Journal of Psychiatry* **170**:2–5.

Brown S, Birtwhistle J, Rowe L, Thomson C (1999). The unhealthy lifestyle of people with schizophrenia. *Psychological Medicine* **29**:697–701.

Burns T, Kendrick T (1997). The primary care of patients with schizophrenia. A search for good practice. *British Journal of General Practice* **47**:515–20.

Taylor P J, Gunn J (1999). Homicides by people with mental illness. Myth and reality. *British Journal of Psychiatry* **174**:9–14.

FURTHER READING

Mental Health Act 1983 Code of Practice (1999). Department of Health and Welsh Office: TSO, London.

Schizophrenia: The Forgotten Illness (1997). SANE, London.

Seminars in General Adult Psychiatry Volume 1 (1998). Stein G, Wilkinson G. (eds) Gaskell, Royal College of Psychiatrists, London.

WEBSITES

General Mental Health
www.mentalhealth.com
Extensive and well-informed links.

Schizophrenia.co.uk
www.schizophrenia.co.uk
News, information and discussion on schizophrenia.

SELF-HELP

Making Space★
18b Otley Road, Headlingley, Leeds LS6 3PX
Tel: 0113 2746010

MIND★★
Granta House, 15–19 Broadway, Stratford, London E15 4BQ
Tel: 020 8519 2122 (administration)
    0345 660163 (information line)

Wales MIND Cymru★★
23 St Mary Street, Cardiff CF1 2AA
Tel: 01222 395123 (administration)
    0345 660163 (information line)

National Schizophrenia Fellowship★★
28 Castle Street, Kingston upon Thames, Surrey KT1 1SS
Tel: 020 8974 6814 (advice line)
Website: www.nsf.org.uk

Sainsbury Centre for Mental Health★
134–138 Borough High Street, London SE1 1LB
Tel: 020 7403 8790 (information line)
Website: www.sainsburycentre.org.uk

SANE★
199–205 Marylebone Road, London NW1 5QP
Tel: 020 7724 6520

Schizophrenia Association of Great Britain★
Bryn Hyfryd, The Crescent, Bangor, Gwynedd LL57 2AG
Tel: 01248 354048
Website: www.btinternet.com/~sagb/

Voices Forum★
28 Castle Street, Kingston upon Thames, Surrey KT1 1SS
Tel: 020 8547 3937

Mental Health Helpline★
Tel: 0345 660606

Saneline National★
Tel: 0345 678000

★ Provides information and support for users and carers
★★ Provides local services for people with serious mental illness

chapter 4

The problem drinker

IN THIS CHAPTER

- Recognizing the problem drinker.
- Brief interventions for the problem drinker.
- Coping with the dependent drinker.
- Safe community detoxification.

EPIDEMIOLOGY

Table 4.1. Epidemiology of alcohol misuse

GP list size 2000
Alcohol above recommended level	320 men	120 women
Harmful levels of alcohol	80 men	16 women

Risk factors: males, drug misuse, genetic, certain occupations

Risk of non-addictive mental disorder: 1/3

Suicide:	x5 men	x18 women
Other violent death:	x4 men	x21 women

Approximately 90% of the population drink alcohol regularly. Between 1950 and 1970, sales of alcohol doubled and the price of alcoholic drinks in real terms has been falling. It has been estimated that alcohol is responsible for 28 000 deaths in England and Wales each year, and one-third of motorists killed on the road are above the legal alcohol limit.

DEFINITION

The drinking patterns of the adult population are shown in Figure 4.1. Three patterns of drinking cause concern:

- Hazardous drinking is consumption above recommended levels but without objective evidence of alcohol related damage.
- Harmful drinking – consumption causing harm.
- Alcohol dependence.

These are important distinctions with implications for both recognition and appropriate management.

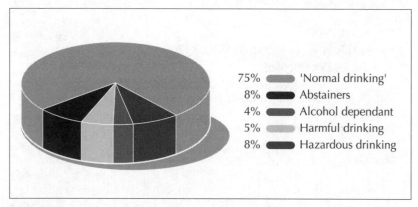

75%	'Normal drinking'
8%	Abstainers
4%	Alcohol dependant
5%	Harmful drinking
8%	Hazardous drinking

Figure 4.1. Drinking patterns in the UK adult population (Chick *et al.*, 1997).

Table 4.2. Definition of levels of alcohol abuse from *Sensible Drinking: the Report of an Inter-departmental Working Group* (1995)

Hazardous alcohol intake
- Men: 3–7 drinks almost every day or 7 or more drinks at least 3 times a week
- Women: 2–5 drinks almost every day or 5 or more drinks at least 3 times a week

Harmful alcohol use (ICD-10)
- Clear evidence that the substance use is responsible for (or is substantially contributing to) physical or psychological harm
- The nature of the harm is clearly identifiable and specified
- The pattern of use has persisted for at least 1 month or has occurred repeatedly within the 12-month period
- The subject does not fulfil criteria for alcohol dependence

Alcohol dependence (at least three items required) (ICD-10)
- Strong desire or sense of compulsion to take the substance
- Impaired capacity to control substance-taking behaviour in terms of onset, termination or levels of use
- Physiological withdrawal state when substance use is reduced or stopped, or use of the substance to relieve or avoid withdrawal symptoms
- Evidence of tolerance to the effects of the substance
- Other pleasures or interests being given up or reduced because of the substance use
- Persistent substance use despite clear evidence of harmful consequences

It is now recognized that there is a J-shaped relationship between intake and mortality. The lowest mortality is seen in those with a small intake, with mortality rising above about 4 units per day. Women are considered to be more susceptible to the harmful effects. Practitioners should be cautious about recommending an increase in drinking given that:

- The mortality data relates to those over 40.
- Individual sensitivity varies.
- There may be harmful behavioural consequences resulting from this advice.

HAZARDOUS AND HARMFUL DRINKERS

✓ Recognition.
✓ Role of blood tests.
✓ Brief intervention.
✓ Interview techniques.

RECOGNITION

Most GPs will be familiar with a number of their patients with alcohol problems. In particular, those who seek help, those who fall foul of the law or those who are brought to the GP's attention by members of their family. These, however, represent the severe end of the spectrum of alcohol consumption and GPs probably remain unaware of three-quarters of hazardous and harmful drinkers.

Patients may be identified opportunistically using sensitive open questions. There are particular opportunities when these questions are more acceptable, e.g. during new patient checks, well-person clinics and the over 75s health check. It is worthwhile asking about alcohol when seeing patients for chronic conditions associated with alcohol use, e.g. hypertension or ischaemic heart disease (IHD). Some occupations are recognized to carry an increased risk of alcohol abuse: barmen, chefs, salesmen, entertainers and seamen.

Some advocate more formal screening and most GPs will be familiar with the CAGE questionnaire (Table 4.3), which works well in outpatients but is not reliable in primary care.

The AUDIT questionnaire (Table 4.4, overleaf) has been validated in primary care but is more complex to administer (Picinelli *et al.*, 1997). If 100 men and women primary care attenders were screened using the AUDIT questionnaire, then 46 potential heavy drinkers (above national safe limits) would be identified of whom 10 would be false positives. An AUDIT-PC version using only items 1, 2, 4, 5 and 10 has almost the same predictive value as the full version. A score of more than 5 on the AUDIT-PC has a positive predictive value of 40% and a negative predictive value of 95% (Aertgerts *et al.*, 2001).

Table 4.3. CAGE questionnaire

Have you ever felt you should **C**ut down on your drinking?

Have people **A**nnoyed you by criticizing your drinking?

Have you ever felt bad or **G**uilty about drinking?

Have you ever taken a drink first thing in the morning (**E**ye-opener) to steady your nerves or get rid of a hangover?

The CAGE questions are not helpful for those patients who deny there is a problem. The questions are more likely to be effective when used in an open way, e.g. 'I always ask everyone about drinking – it can be helpful to talk about drinking without feeling got at. Tell me have you ever been worried about your drinking? Ever? In any way? I mean has it lead to rows or troubles at home or at work? Health troubles? Ever thought you ought to cut down? Anyone criticized your drinking?'

(Edwards *et al.*, 1997)

Table 4.4. AUDIT (Alcohol Use Disorders Identification Test)

One unit of alcohol is: half a pint of average strength beer/lager, or 1 glass of wine, or 1 single measure of spirits.

Note: a can of high-strength beer or lager may contain 3–4 units.

1 How often do you have a drink containing alcohol? ☐
(0) Never   (1) Monthly or less   (2) 2–4 times a month
(3) 2–3 times a week   (4) 4 or more times a week

2 How many units of alcohol do you drink on a typical day ☐
when you are drinking?
(0) 1 or 2   (1) 3 or 4   (2) 5 or 6
(3) 7, 8 or 9   (4) 10 or more

3 How often do you have 6 or more units of alcohol on one ☐
occasion?
(0) Never   (1) Less than monthly   (2) Monthly
(3) Weekly   (4) Daily or almost daily

4 How often during the last year have you found that you ☐
were not able to stop drinking once you had started?
(0) Never   (1) Less than monthly   (2) Monthly
(3) Weekly   (4) Daily or almost daily

5 How often during the last year have you failed to do ☐
what was normally expected of you because of drinking?
(0) Never   (1) Less than monthly   (2) Monthly
(3) Weekly   (4) Daily or almost daily

6 How often during the last year have you needed a first drink inthe morning to get yourself going after a heavy drinking session?

(0) Never   (1) Less than monthly   (2) Monthly
(3) Weekly   (4) Daily or almost daily

☐

7 How often during the last year have you had a feeling of guilt or remorse after drinking?

(0) Never   (1) Less than monthly   (2) Monthly
(3) Weekly   (4) Daily or almost daily

☐

8 How often during the last year have you been unable to rememberwhat happened the night before because you had been drinking?

(0) Never   (1) Less than monthly   (2) Monthly
(3) Weekly   (4) Daily or almost daily

☐

9 Have you or someone else been injured as a result of your drinking?

(0) No   (2) Yes but not in the last year
(4) Yes, during the last year

☐

10 Has a relative or friend or doctor or another health worker been concerned about your drinking or suggested you cut down?

(0) No   (2) Yes but not in the last year
(4) Yes, during the last year

☐

Record the total of specific items here
If the total is over 8, alcohol use disorder is very likely

☐

Table 4.5. Trauma questionnaire

In the past 5 years:
Have you had any fractures or dislocations to your bones or joints?
Have you been injured in a road traffic accident?
Have you injured your head?
Have you been injured in a fight or an assault?

Final question asked by the physician if an affirmative answer to one or more of the above:
Have you been injured while or after consuming alcoholic drinks?

A further approach to increased recognition was adopted in a Canadian trial by pre-screening primary care attenders with a 'Trauma questionnaire' (Table 4.5). Only those answering 'yes' to one or more trauma questions were brought to the attention of their physician for further enquiries. All patients answering positively to two questions and those answering positively to the one about alcohol were further questioned about alcohol consumption. One in seven of patients were subsequently asked about alcohol use and the method identified 62–85% of the expected problem drinkers in the population (Israel *et al.*, 1996).

ROLE OF BLOOD TESTS

Blood tests may be abnormal in heavy drinkers, but their sensitivity and specificity are too low to be useful for screening (Chick *et al.*, 1981). Blood tests have a role in identifying when the line has been crossed between hazardous and harmful drinking, and they can be used to follow up progress of those on treatment programmes.

- GGT (gamma-glutamyltransferase): raised in about 60% of people drinking more than 56 units/week (probably less for women). False positives include liver disease of other causes, and anticonvulsants. Usually normalizes after 2–3 weeks of abstinence.
- MCV (mean corpuscular volume): raised in about 30% of people drinking more than 56 units/week (probably less for women). False positives include B_{12} and folate deficiency, other liver disease, haematological malignancy, hypothyroidism, drug effects. It takes 1–3 months of abstinence to return to baseline.
- CDT (carbohydrate deficient transferin): raised in 60–80% people drinking more than 56 units/week. Not affected by prescribed drugs or common medical disorders. Not yet routinely available.

(UK Alcohol Forum, 1997)

GPs and practice nurses underestimate the amount patients drink because they are often unaware of the alcohol content of drinks. A simple formula gives units of alcohol:

$$\text{Units} = \frac{\text{volume (ml)} \times \% \text{ abv (alcohol by volume)}}{1000}$$

Table 4.6. Alcohol content of common drinks

	Units
10 pints of lager (Stella Artois) 5.2% abv	30
10 pints of bitter (Boddingtons) 3.8% abv	22
4 bottles of red wine 12% abv (70 cl size)	36
1 bottle of gin 37.5% abv (70 cl size)	26
10 cans of Diamond White cider 8.4% abv (440 ml size)	37

(Webster-Harris *et al.*, 2001)

BRIEF INTERVENTIONS IN PRIMARY CARE

It is now established that a brief intervention offered at primary care level to hazardous drinkers is likely to be effective, with about one-quarter of individuals reporting reduced alcohol consumption following intervention (Effective Healthcare, 1993). It is less clear how reducing alcohol consumption by this approach translates into health gain for the population.

SUGGESTED CONTENT OF A BRIEF INTERVENTION

Information: personalized information regarding safe levels.

Advice: how to cut down on drinking including simple behavioural measures, e.g.:

- Counting the number of drinks and timing how long it takes to finish; put the glass down between drinking.
- Sipping rather than gulping.
- Using non-alcoholic spacers, e.g buy yourself a non-alcoholic drink when it is 'your round'.
- Eating before and during drinking (this reduces appetite and slows alcohol absorption).
- Avoid salty food whilst drinking (it is a thirst stimulant).
- Use low alcohol drinks.
- Have drink free days.

Reinforcement: reinforce upper safe limits of consumption.

Personal rules: set your own rules to reinforce the behavioural approach.

Self monitoring: use a drink diary to monitor the success of changes.

Brief counselling:
- Motivational enhancement.
- Identification of high-risk situations.
- Identification of alternative activities and interests.

(Adapted from *Medicine*, 1999)

INTERVIEW TECHNIQUES

Brief counselling using a simple mnemonic FRAMES (Feedback, Responsibility, Advice, Menu of options, Empathy and Self-efficacy) could be feasibly applied during a routine primary care consultation (Table 4.7).

Table 4.7. Counselling using FRAMES

Feedback
'Have you considered that your difficulties (e.g. sexual) may be related to use of alcohol?'

Responsibility
'Only you can decide. Why don't you see what happens if you cut down for a couple of weeks?'

Advice
'I recommend that you stop drinking and see if that improves the situation.'

Menu of options
'I appreciate you may not be able to manage this but if you find it hard going then our counsellor may be able to help. We could also arrange for you to attend the local self-help group.'

Empathy
'I know this must be hard for you because the wine helps you to relax and I am concerned by the amount of stress in your life.'

Self-efficacy
'Considering this has been going on such a long time it's good that you have asked for help. Your own determination will help you get through.'

CASE STUDY: JOE

Joe, his wife and two small children were newly registered with the practice. He was a sales representative and regularly entertained clients for lunch. At his registration health check he revealed that he was consuming an average of 40 units of alcohol a week. He was not aware of any adverse effects and considered his intake to be normal as part of his job. The practice nurse gave him an information leaflet.

Joe presented 6 months later following a fall in which he had fractured his thumb. Dr Smith asked him again about his alcohol consumption. It turned out he had not reduced his intake and, if anything, it had increased as he had joined a local snooker club where he spent two evenings each week. He had slipped on his way home and admitted to having had 'one or two' drinks. Dr Smith suggested an upper limit for his weekly consumption and suggested ways he could reduce his intake at lunchtimes without being conspicuous. Joe recognized that his evenings out had become associated with drinking and agreed to limit himself to one drink. When he was seen prior to returning to work the limits were re-emphasized. One year later whilst his GP was seeing his wife on a postnatal visit, Joe mentioned that he had reduced his alcohol consumption and felt better for it, he had since been promoted.

Lessons from the case study
■ Alcohol problems in a high-risk occupation presenting with trauma.
■ Integration of a brief intervention into routine health care:
  – personalized information,
  – negotiated simple behavioural modification,
  – re-emphasis of limits.

Alcohol dependence

Most practitioners will not have problems identifying patients with alcohol dependence – they may present directly seeking help or with physical ailments directly attributable to alcohol intoxication. Alcohol dependence should be considered as a chronic relapsing disease, not unlike diabetes or IHD. It is now widely recognized that successful treatment for a myocardial infarction does not stop at the time of hospital discharge and in the same way successful treatment of alcohol dependency does not stop after successful detoxification. For the majority of patients a relapsing course is the norm and should not be considered a treatment failure.

✓ Prognosis.
✓ Detoxification.
✓ Relapse prevention.
✓ When to refer.

Prognosis

There are few long-term prospective studies and available data are sparse. Mortality rates for those who have been in contact with specialist clinics are consistently higher than for the general population. Causes of death are frequently alcohol related, with heart disease more common in older males. Cirrhosis, neoplasms and violent deaths are more common in all age groups.

Treatment for alcohol addiction is successful in the short term, with half of those treated showing a 50% reduction in use after 6 months, but only 20–50% of patients remain abstinent during the first year. Long-term remission rates vary widely from 21–80%. Some studies indicate that there is a spontaneous remission rate of up to 65% without professional help. Patients who comply with education, medication and counselling have a better outlook, but compliance is notoriously poors. Drinking levels prior to treatment are weak predictors of long-term remission, but are related to subsequent ill health and mortality. Once remission is secured, then those who achieve 5 years' abstinence have a dramatically reduced relapse rate compared to those with 1 or 2 years (Taylor, 1994).

PREDICTORS OF POOR COMPLIANCE AND RELAPSE

- Low socio-economic status.
- Co-morbid psychiatric conditions.
- Lack of family or social support.

(O'Brien and Mclellan, 1996)

MANAGEMENT IN PRIMARY CARE

The approach to management will be determined to some extent by the presentation of the patient, and whether they are seeking help and willing to comply with strategies to reduce damage from alcohol. There is a debate whether complete abstinence or a reduction in alcohol intake should be the goal of treatment. GPs will need a working knowledge of support services available in their area and an established pathway of care. Strategies will include community detoxification, inpatient detoxification, referral to residential programmes and maintenance programmes. In addition, primary care teams may be involved in supporting the family of those with alcohol dependence.

DETOXIFICATION

The decision regarding community or inpatient detoxification will be made with due regard to available services, the situation of the patient and the severity of withdrawal syndromes. These syndromes may be categorized into mild, intermediate and major. There is no way of predicting the severity of a withdrawal reaction, and marked variation may occur even within one patient in subsequent episodes. Caution should be exercised when the patient gives a history of a previous major reaction.

Mild withdrawal

Symptoms occur within a few hours of withdrawal, and consist of apprehension, weakness, sweating, irritability, insomnia and tremor. Recovery is usual in 24–72 hours. Most practitioners will be familiar with the mild withdrawal syndrome and should have a locally agreed strategy for community detoxification. Benzodiazepines are recommended with a short-reducing course employed to control symptoms. Chlordiazepoxide at an initial dose of 20 mg four times a day, over 48 hours, reducing over 10 days, is a common regime. It is recommended that multivitamin preparations containing at least 200 mg of thiamine daily are co-prescribed. Chlormethiazole is not recommended in the community due to a potentially fatal interaction with alcohol. Many patients refer to these symptoms as 'DTs', although this is a misnomer as delirium tremens represents a serious and potentially fatal withdrawal reaction for which admission is mandatory.

Intermediate withdrawal

In addition to the above, patients may develop hallucinations, convulsions and, rarely, dysrhythmias.

Major withdrawal (delirium tremens)

Major withdrawal symptoms are severe agitation, confusion, delusions, gross tremor, tachycardia and sweating. Extreme fear may lead to aggressive, destructive or suicidal behaviour. These features are seen within 3 days after cessation of alcohol and may last 3–7 days. With supportive treatment, mortality is about 1%; death is usually from cardiovascular collapse or infection. Patients should be sent into hospital as an emergency.

Table 4.8. Indications for inpatient assisted withdrawal

- History of withdrawal seizures
- Signs of delirium
- Severe vomiting
- Risk of self-harm
- Lack of home support
- Severe dependency and unwilling to be seen daily
- Previous failure of community detoxification
- Uncontrollable withdrawal symptoms
- Acute physical illness
- Poly-substance abuse
- Home environment is unsupportive of abstinence

(UK Alcohol Forum, 1997)

SELECTING FOR COMMUNITY DETOXIFICATION

There is good evidence that assisted withdrawal and treatment in the community is effective. Many patients can be detoxified safely and effectively at home, but only those with mild withdrawal reactions are suitable. Table 4.8 sets out the indicators for inpatient assisted withdrawal.

FAMILY SUPPORT

Family doctors will be familiar with the potentially devastating effects on the family associated with a problem drinker. Partners of drinkers may seek help either for themselves or their spouse. Alcohol and drug services often concentrate on those using alcohol or drugs potentially neglecting family members. Relatives are often under stress and may themselves suffer harmful effects on mental or physical health. One model of family response to alcohol abuse, the stress-coping model, recognizes that coping strategies may compound the problem by supporting, colluding or refusing to challenge risky behaviour. GPs may help by providing support and encouragement to challenge adverse coping strategies, as well as appropriate referral to local agencies.

RELAPSE PREVENTION

Recognizing that alcohol abuse is a chronic relapsing disease and that probably only half of patients will remain abstinent from alcohol in the first year following acute alcohol detoxification, what can the primary health care team do to help in relapse prevention and management? Friedman *et al.* (1998) outline a menu of potential options for which they admit there is little research evidence regarding their effectiveness (Table 4.9). Predominant precipitants of relapse are negative affective states, such as anger, frustration, boredom, fatigue and loneliness. The 12-step recovery groups use the acronym HALT: do not get Hungry, Angry, Lonely or Tired. There may be also be situational triggers, e.g. favoured bars or having ready cash. Helping patients recognize environmental and situational triggers may be helpful. Patients should avoid 'testing' themselves in these situations early in their recovery. The authors suggest developing a plan to cope with episodes of relapse. Patients who return to drink may feel guilt and despair and, feeling there is nothing to lose, indulge in a serious binge. The patient should be encouraged to see beyond the initial guilt and even to try and learn from the relapse. An individual response to relapse should be negotiated, limiting use and seeking help immediately.

Table 4.9. Relapse prevention strategies in primary care

- Identify patients in recovery
- Establish a supportive patient–physician relationship
- Schedule regular follow-up
- Use family support
- Facilitate involvement in self-help groups
- Help recovering patients recognize and manage relapse precipitants and craving
- Develop a plan to cope with potential relapse
- Facilitate positive lifestyle changes
- Manage depression, anxiety and other co-morbid conditions
- Consider adjunctive medication
- Collaborate with addiction speciality professionals

(Adapted from Friedman *et al.*, 1998)

ANXIETY AND DEPRESSION IN ALCOHOL DEPENDENCE

Stopping drinking is the critical intervention. Patients need to be aware that alcohol has a depressant effect, disrupts sleep, and withdrawal effects may mimic anxiety. If a trial of antidepressants is considered, avoid TCAs because they potentiate the action of alcohol and are dangerous in overdose. If available a psychological intervention should be considered as first line, looking at drinking together with family, social and cognitive factors.

WHEN TO REFER

There are four indications for referral:

- *Access to specialist services*, e.g. community alcohol teams considering disulfiram or acamprosate treatment.
- *Co-morbidity:* there is a high level of physical and psychiatric co-morbidity in patients with an alcohol problem. Patients with serious medical complications need medical and, possibly, psychiatric referral (depending on the configuration of local services). Patients with severe mental illness (psychoses) and an alcohol problem should be in the care of specialist services.
- *Detoxification* in high-risk individuals.
- *Withdrawal:* intermediate or severe withdrawal syndrome.

WHAT TO EXPECT FROM SECONDARY CARE

Management
- Detoxification.
- Drug therapies to prevent relapse.

Disulfiram
Disulfiram blocks acetaldehyde breakdown. Alcohol intake leads to acetaldehyde accumulation with flushing, headaches, palpitations, nausea and vomiting. Large doses of alcohol may precipitate a fatal cardiovascular collapse.

Suitable patients are those who need extra help in remaining abstinent, particularly those for whom there are serious social consequences of a relapse. It is effective only if taken regularly (helped by third-party supervision).

Acamprosate

Acamprosate reduces the risk of relapse following detoxification. It reduces the urge to drink by stimulating central gamma-aminobutyric acid (GABA)-ergic inhibitory neurotransmission. It is started immediately after detoxification, continued for a year and used only as part of a treatment package involving counselling support.

CASE STUDY: HARRY

I first met Harry when he moved in to the nearby single man's shelter. He was an alcoholic and had been discharged from the army through drink. He suffered from a chronic anxiety disorder and was also depressed. He was consuming 80 units weekly and wanted to stop; without drug support he suffered agitation and a marked tremor. He had been successfully detoxified in the community in the past, and although he lived alone we negotiated a withdrawal schedule. The detoxification was successful and although he continued to drink it was at a much reduced level. The depression responded to treatment and when he was given a council flat he became quite buoyant.

Harry presented 1 year later having relapsed. He recognized the precipitant had been a stressful part-time job leading to low mood. Following a further successful community detoxification, we discussed early recognition of relapse and avoidance of situations which he associated with drink. He kept a 'craving diary' and noted that his worst times were when he was tired and hungry and when he had ready cash. We discussed avoidance of these triggers and a strategy of diverting himself with television. I explained that such cravings are uncomfortable, but a normal feature of recovery. They may last minutes or hours and should not lead to shame.

Harry attended alcoholics anonymous and, for a while, all was well. He defaulted from follow up and I next saw him following a haematemesis. He had portal congestion and a duodenal ulcer. He had been drinking again and had not contacted me through guilt despite our earlier discussion. He remained alcohol free after discharge and saw me for medication review over the next 2 years. He was noted to have thrombocytopenia on a blood film, and the haematologist put this down to probable chronic liver disease. He was referred to the local gastroenterologist, but 6 months later he had not yet been seen and asked for an urgent visit. He was in a bad way with a prominent flapping tremor and gross ascites. He had not eaten for 2 days because he could not walk and had no local family or friends to help out. I arranged an admission the same day, but he died 1 week later from alcoholic cirrhosis and liver failure.

Lessons from the case study

- Even those with a chronic problem may benefit from help.
- The presence of poor prognostic markers:
  - single male,
  - poor social support,
  - severe chronic problem.
- Community detoxification is possible even in the chronic drinker.
- Relapse after detoxification is almost inevitable and should not be regarded as therapeutic failure.
- Treatment of co-morbid conditions aids recovery.
- Complete abstinence may be an unrealistic goal.
- Identify triggers for relapse and strategies for avoidance.
- Encourage early presentation following relapse.
- Involve appropriate outside agencies.

REFERENCES

Aertgeert SB, Bunting XF, Ansoms S, Feverly J (2001). Screening properties of questionnaires and laboratory tests for the detection of alcohol abuse or dependence in the general practice population. *British Journal of General Practice* **51**:206–17.

Chick J, Kreitman N, Plant M (1981). Mean cell volume and gamma-glutamyl-transpeptidase as markers of drinking in working men. *Lancet* **1(8232)**:1249–51.

Chick J, Godfrey C, Hore B, Marshall EJ, Peters T (1997). *Alcohol Dependence: A Clinical Problem.* Mosby-Wolfe, London.

Edwards G, Marshall E, Cook C (1997). *The Treatment of Drinking Problems.* Cambridge University Press, Cambridge.

Effective Health Care (1993). *Brief Interventions and Alcohol Use.* University of Leeds, Leeds.

Friedman P, Saitz R, Samet J (1998). Management of adults recovering from alcohol or other drug problems. *Journal of the American Medical Association* **279**:1227–31.

Israel Y, Hollander O, Sanchez-Craig M, Booker S, Miller V, Gingrich R, Rankin J (1996). Screening for problem drinking and counseling by the primary care physician-nurse team. *Alcoholism: Clinical and Experimental Research* **20**:1443–9.

Medicine (1999). 27(2). The Medicine Publishing Company, Abingdon.

O'Brien CP, Mclellan AT (1996). Myths about the treatment of addiction. *Lancet* **347**:237–40.

Piccinelli M, Tessari E, Bortolomasi M, Piasere O, Semenzin M, Garzotto N, Tansella M (1997). Efficacy of the alcohol use disorders identification test as a screening tool for hazardous alcohol intake and related disorders in primary care: a validity study [see comments]. *British Medical Journal* **314(7078)**:420–4.

Sensible Drinking: the Report of an Inter-departmental Working Group (1995). HMSO, London.

Taylor C (1994). What happens over the long-term? *British Medical Bulletin* **50**:50–66.

UK Alcohol Forum (1997). *Guidelines for the management of alcohol problems in primary care and general psychiatry.* Tangent Medical Education.

Webster-Harris PJ, Barton AG, Barton SM, Anderson SD (2001). General practitioners and practice nurses knowledge of how much patients should and do drink. *British Journal of General Practice* **51**:218–20.

FURTHER READING

Anon (2000). Managing the heavy drinker in primary care. *Drugs and Therapeutics Bulletin* **38**:60–64.

WEBSITES

Medical Council on Alcoholism
www.medicouncilalsol.demon.co.uk
Provides information and advice about alcohol problems.

Habit Smart Web (Addictions)
www.habitsmart.com
Self-scoring alcohol questionnaire, advice and information.

SELF-HELP

Alcohol Concern
Waterbridge House, 32–36 Loman Street, London SE1 0EE
Tel: 020 7928 7377
Website: www.alcoholconcern.org.uk
Help and information about alcohol problems.

Alcoholics Anonymous
PO Box 1, Stonebrow House, Stonebrow, York YO1 2NJ
Tel: 01904 644026 (administration)
     020 7352 3001 (helpline)
Website: www.alcoholics-anonymous.org
Voluntary fellowship of men and women who share their experience, strength
and hope that they may solve their common problems and help others to recover
from alcoholism.

A1-Anon Family Groups
61 Great Dover Street, London SE1 4YF
Helpline: 020 7403 0888 (24 hours)
Website: www.hexnet.co.uk/a1anon/
Provides help and support for relatives and friends of alcoholics. Alateen, a part of
A1-Anon, is for teenagers affected by a drinking problem of a relative or close friend.

Drinkline (National Alcohol Helpline)
Helpline: 0500 801 802
Provides information and advice to callers worried about their own drinking,
support for family and friends of people who are drinking and advises callers on
where to go for help.

Turning Point
New Loom House, 101 Backchurch Lane, London E1 1LU
Tel: 020 7702 2300
Website: www.turning-point.co.uk
Helps anyone with problems relating to drink and drug misuse, mental health
problems or learning disabilities, including family and friends.

chapter 5

The forgetful and confused patient

IN THIS CHAPTER

- Recognizing early dementia.
- Simple screening for dementia.
- Distinguishing dementia from depression.
- Dementia and the law: driving, the Mental Health Act, power of attorney.
- Management of behavioural disturbance.
- Drugs for Alzheimer's disease.

INTRODUCTION

The major mental illnesses of the elderly are dementia, delirium and depression. Although it is important to distinguish between these three disorders, there is often an overlap which may muddy the diagnostic waters.

EPIDEMIOLOGY

Approximately 5% of the population over 65 has dementia. Key epidemiological facts are shown in Table 5.1 (overleaf).

Delirium or an acute confusional state has a prevalence of at least 5% in general hospitals but no figures are available for community prevalence

Table 5.1. Epidemiology of dementia

- Prevalence increases with age (approximately doubling each 5 years):
  - 2% age 65–70
  - 20% age 80+
- Equal prevalence in men and women
- Risk factors:
  - family history
  - family history of Down's syndrome or Parkinson's disease
  - head injury
  - depression
  - maternal age 40+
- Causes of dementia:
  - Alzheimer's disease 50%
  - vascular 20%
  - Lewy body 15%

– reflecting its transient nature and high mortality. Patients with dementia are at increased risk of delirium and an episode of delirium may be the factor which brings a dementing process to light.

RECOGNITION AND DIAGNOSIS

- ✓ Clinical features of dementia.
- ✓ Testing for cognitive impairment.
- ✓ Physical investigations.
- ✓ Differential diagnosis:
  - Lewy body dementia,
  - depression,
  - confusional states.

Dementia is often equated with loss of memory. However, the complaint of subjective memory impairment is a poor indicator of dementia. Subjective memory impairment correlates more with depression than dementia. Informant reports of memory loss, together with symptoms of altered functioning, are likely pointers to dementia. Dementia is more than memory impairment, other important features are listed below:

CLINICAL FEATURES OF DEMENTIA

- Decline in intellectual functioning (memory, thinking and judgement).
- Decline in everyday functioning (dressing, washing, cooking).
- Loss of emotional control.
- Behavioural changes: apathy or agitation.
- Dysphasia and dyspraxia.

Until recently, there was little incentive for the GP to make an early diagnosis of dementia in that there were no active treatments available. However, the availability of antidementia drugs has changed this. These drugs are most effective in the early stages of the illness.

INITIAL RECOGNITION

The presence of the clinical symptoms listed above should alert the GP to the possibility of cognitive impairment. Patients rarely seek medical attention for the symptoms of dementia, and even family members often attribute symptoms to normal ageing.

Normal ageing is associated with a slowing of cognitive performance, but not a reduction in capability. However, ageing is associated with concurrent illnesses and pharmacological treatments that reduce cognition.

It is vital to talk with an informant as part of making or excluding a diagnosis of dementia.

Testing for cognitive impairment

Although there is little evidence supporting routine screening for dementia, testing for cognitive impairment in selected patients may assist in making a diagnosis. The mini mental state examination (MMSE) (Folstein *et al.*, 1975) is widely used to detect cognitive impairment. It takes on average about 10 minutes to administer. An arbitrary cut off at 25 out of 30 separates possible cognitive from no cognitive impairment. This will be influenced by premorbid educational status. One of the important uses of the mini mental state examination is that the scores are linked to the current National Institute for Clinical Excellence (NICE) guidelines for the use of drugs for the treatment of Alzheimer's disease (see page 137).

The full mini mental state examination is listed in Table 5.2.

Table 5.2. The mini mental state examination

Date:

Orientation
1 Day................ 2 Date................ 3 Month................ 4 Year................ 5 *Season................
*Allow flexibility when season changes, e.g. March = winter/spring, June = spring/summer

6 Number.......... 7 Address............. 8 Town/city............. 9 County............ 10. Country.............
(e.g. ward/house number, hospital/street)

Maximum 10 points........./10

Registration
11 Name three objects (e.g. apple, table, penny), taking 1 second to say each clearly. Ask the patient to repeat them until all three are repeated (maximum five attempts). Score 1 for each correct answer.

Maximum 3 points........../3

Concentration
12 Spell 'WORLD' backwards. Score 1 point for each letter in the correct order, even if partly incorrect sequence of omissions, e.g. DROW scores 3 points, as does DLORW

Maximum 5 points........../5

Recall
13 Ask for the names of the three objects registered earlier.

Maximum 3 points........../3

Praxis
14 Three-stage command. Say, 'I am going to hand you a piece of paper, when I do so, please take it with your right hand, fold it in half with BOTH hands and place it on your lap.' Do not repeat the instructions or prompt. Score a move as correct only if it takes place in the right sequence; give 1 point for each correct move.

Maximum 3 points........../3

Articulation
15 Ask to repeat the following, 'No ifs, ands or buts.'

Maximum 1 point.............../1

Naming
16 Point to (a) a watch and (b) a pen/pencil, and ask to name each one as you point.

Maximum 2 points.........../2

Comprehension
17 Ask, 'Please can you read this and do what I say.' If it cannot be read, it is acceptable to read it out to the person.

Maximum 1 point.............../1

Close your eyes

Copying
18 Ask, 'Please can you copy this design in the space beside it' (point to it). Each pentagon should have five sides and five corners.

Maximum 1 point.............../1

Writing
19 Please write a sentence in the space below (point to bottom of sheet). The sentence should make sense and be grammatically correct, but spelling mistakes can be ignored.

Maximum 1 point................./1

Total.............../30

Briefer tests of cognitive function can be used to pick out patients with an increased risk of dementia (Siu, 1991). Four of these are set out below.

Orientation to day

What day is it today?

This question has high specificity (92%) but a low sensitivity (53%) in predicting cognitive impairment. If the patient gets the day wrong it greatly increases the probability of cognitive impairment, getting the day correct, however, does not exclude dementia. Another way of looking at screening results is to use the likelihood ratios:

> Orientation to day has a likelihood ratio of 0.5.
> Disorientation to day has a likelihood ratio of 6:3.

Likelihood ratios can be used to convert pre-test probabilities into post-test probabilities. The likelihood ratio for a positive test result is the likelihood that a positive test comes from a person with the disorder rather than one without. When using likelihood ratios to convert pre-test probabilities to post-test probabilities use the nomogram in Streiner and Geddes (1998).

The results of a test in predicting a disorder depend on the prevalence of the disorder in the population tested. The post-test possibilities of dementia being present in three scenarios are set out below:

	Likelihood ratio	*Patient age 70* Prevalence of dementia 2%	*Patient age 85* Prevalence of dementia 25%	*Suspected dementia* Prevalence of dementia 50%
Day correct	0.5	1%	14%	33%
Day incorrect	6.3	11%	68%	86%

Thus if all patients aged 85 are screened for dementia, getting the day correct reduces the chance of dementia from 25% to 14%. If we assume that when the GP suspects dementia he/she is right 50% of the time, getting the day correct reduces the chance to 33%, whereas getting the day incorrect increases the probability to 86%.

Recall of three items

> I would like you to repeat back to me the following three items: apple, penny, table. The patient repeats.
>
> I am going to ask you to remember those three items in 5 minutes.
>
> Ask again after 5 minutes – use the time in between to continue the consultation.

The inability to recall at least two out of three items affects the probability of dementia being present as shown:

	Likelihood ratio	*Patient age 70* Prevalence of dementia 2%	*Patient age 85* Prevalence of dementia 25%	*Suspected dementia* Prevalence of dementia 50%
Recall of 2 or 3 items	0.5	1%	14%	33%
Recall of 0 or 1 items	3.1	6%	51%	76%

Serial sevens

I would like you to take 7 away from 100 and keep taking 7 from your answer.

Subtracting sevens backwards from 100 to 79 has a low specificity, but a high sensitivity (the reverse of orientation to day). Thus the ability to do serial sevens is good at ruling out dementia, but an inability to do serial sevens stems from many causes.

	Likelihood ratio	*Patient age 70* Prevalence of dementia 2%	*Patient age 85* Prevalence of dementia 25%	*Suspected dementia* Prevalence of dementia 50%
Correct	0.06	0.1%	2%	6%
Incorrect	1.9	4%	39%	65%

Clock drawing

Please draw a clock face with the numbers and hands.

	Likelihood ratio	*Patient age 70* Prevalence of dementia 2%	*Patient age 85* Prevalence of dementia 25%	*Suspected dementia* Prevalence of dementia 50%
Very abnormal	24	32%	89%	96%
Almost normal	0.8	2%	21%	44%
Normal	0.2	0.4%	6%	17%

Table 5.3. Shortened mini mental state examination to screen for dementia

	Likelihood ratios	
	Correct	Incorrect
Orientation to day	0.6	10.2
Spell word 'WORLD' backwards	0.5	2.2
Recall three words (correct is 2 or 3)	0.4	2.8
Write a sentence	0.9	2.8

(Wind *et al.*, 1997)

It can be seen that fairly quick tests of cognitive function make a considerable difference to the probability of dementia being present. A shortened screen for dementia picking out key items from the mini mental state examination is given in Table 5.3. This has been recommended for use in primary care (Eccles *et al.*, 1998).

The astute reader will notice slightly difference likelihood ratios in the table above from those given earlier in the chapter. This reflects data drawn from different patient samples.

Assessing functional impairment

Functional impairment should be assessed alongside intellectual impairment. Patients with dementia lose social skills. Four activities of daily living are significantly associated with cognitive impairment:

- Managing medication.
- Using the telephone.
- Coping with a budget.
- Using transportation.

Ask an informant as well as the patient about coping in these areas.

Physical screening in dementia patients

The importance of excluding treatable causes haunts psychiatry. In the past, the emphasis has been on excluding physical causes, however rare and unlikely, at the expense of treating psychological disorders in physical conditions, however common. A very small proportion of people with dementia have an underlying abnormality which, when treated, may result in improved cognitive function. Reversible dementias are only found in 1% of elderly patients who are assessed in memory clinics (Walstra *et al.*, 1997). Higher rates of potentially treatable causes are found in younger people and those presenting with a short history of impairment. Brain imaging should be considered in patients with a short and atypical history, or with neurological signs not explained by known cerebrovascular disease.

It is important to be aware that patients with dementia may not complain of common physical symptoms.

Much more common than a treatable cause for dementia is the presence of a superimposed confusional state which does need appropriate investigation and treatment.

PHYSICAL INVESTIGATIONS OF PATIENTS WITH DEMENTIA

- Full blood count and erythrocyte sedimentation rate.
- Biochemical screening including serum, calcium and phosphate.
- Thyroid function.
- Glucose.

Testing for syphilis should be done only if clinically indicated. Overall, the probability of a patient with an abnormal test having neurosyphilis is 2%; a negative test does not rule out the diagnosis (Frank, 1998).

Differential diagnosis of dementia

The differential diagnosis of dementia is a function for secondary care. GPs do need to be aware, however, of Lewy body dementia. Lewy body dementia accounts for approximately 15% of dementias, overlapping with

Alzheimer's disease and dementia associated with Parkinson's disease. In Lewy body dementia, memory impairment may not be an early feature. The clinical symptoms are shown below. A possible diagnosis of Lewy body dementia is made in the presence of dementia and at least one core symptom.

CLINICAL SYMPTOMS OF LEWY BODY TYPE DEMENTIA (% OF CASES)

- Complex visual hallucinations (48%).★
- Fluctuating cognition and clouding of consciousness (81%).★
- Extrapyramidal features (9.5%).★
- Auditory hallucinations (14%).
- Paranoid delusions (57%).
- Falls or collapses (38%).
- Depression (38%).

★ Core symptoms

The importance of Lewy body dementia is that patients have markedly increased sensitivity to typical neuroleptics which should not be prescribed. Atypical neuroleptics may be less likely to cause problems, but should be used only with caution.

Vascular dementia accounts for about 15% of cases of dementia. Clinical features include abrupt onset, stepwise progression and an association with other vascular conditions, particularly strokes and cardiovascular disease.

Distinguishing between dementia and depressive disorder

Depressive disorders may coexist with dementia, the prevalence of depression being 10–40% of patients with dementia. Table 5.4 indicates the features which might enable a clinical differentiation of dementia from depression. Where depression is suspected, it should be treated. There is

Table 5.4. Clinical differentiation of dementia from depression

	Dementia	Depression
Onset	Insidious	Recent (weeks)
Emotion	Shallow, apathetic	Distressed
Subjective memory	Often not complained about	Complaint of cognitive difficulties
Orientation	May be normal, usually impaired for time/place	Usually normal
Answers to specific questions	Confabulation or inadequate responses	Often 'don't know' responses
Dyspraxia, dysphasia	May be present	Not present

good evidence that even in cases where depression coexists with dementia, treatment with antidepressant medication is of value.

Distinguishing between dementia and acute confusional states

Confusional states are acute in onset, fluctuate in intensity and are often worse at night. Orientation is always impaired. Confusional states are often associated with visual and auditory hallucinations, delusional ideas, together with a fearful or aggressive mood. Acute confusional states can be superimposed upon a dementia, and may be the reason that the patient with dementia presents to medical services.

Diogenes syndrome

Diogenes was a Greek philosopher of the fourth century BC. He proposed a self-sufficient way of life disregarding material possessions. The Diogenes syndrome has become applied to cases of 'severe squalor'. Suspicious elderly people are found living in isolated, often filthy and unhygienic, conditions. Such patients merit referral to specialist services for assessment, but only about half are found to be mentally ill.

MANAGEMENT IN PRIMARY CARE

Diagnosis and information for patients and carers

GPs are often reluctant to inform patients and their relatives about the diagnosis or the prognosis of dementia. There are advantages, however, in the early diagnosis and information provision for such patients:

- Allows the patient and family to plan appropriately for the future.
- Allows access to treatments of potential benefit in improving cognitive decline.
- Ensures the patient receives appropriate services and benefits.

Support for carers

- Referral of carers to groups for the provision of support and information about dementia.
- Referral of the patient to respite and day-care services.
- Identifying and treating depressive disorder in carers.
- Advice about legal steps to safeguard finances.

Psychosocial interventions

- Advise the patient to keep up simple exercise to maintain ambulation.
- Advise carers to modulate the environment to reduce stimulation, and that they establish regular routines.
- In conversation, keep sentences short and keep reminding the patient about content.
- Keep the patient orientated – the date, day, lists to do.

(Small *et al.*, 1997)

Drug treatments

- Aspirin 75 mg may reduce the risk of further vascular events for patients with early dementia related to cerebral ischaemia.
- At present, it is recommended that GPs should not initiate treatment with specific antidementia drugs (see page 137).

Driving and dementia

The DVLA must be notified as soon as a diagnosis is made. Driving is permissible in early dementia if there is no significant disorientation in time and place, and there is adequate retention of insight and judgement. An annual medical review will be required.

The GP should advise the patient that they have a condition which requires them to inform the DVLA – this should be documented in the case notes. If the patient does not inform the DVLA and continues to drive, the GP should consider informing the DVLA directly. The DVLA will then contact the patient, but not indicate the source of their information.

THE MANAGEMENT OF BEHAVIOURAL DISTURBANCE

Agitated behaviours: biting, scratching, screaming, pacing

- Check and remedy the cause: Stewart's (1991) mneumonic, five I's:
  - Iatrogenic (drug),
  - Infection (urinary tract infection, pneumonia),
  - Illness (worsening chronic illness, pain),
  - Inconsistency (a recent change in the environment/routine),
  - Is the patient depressed/psychotic?
- Support care givers:
  - define the problem,
  - monitor the problem,
  - simple verbal/non-verbal instructions for carers to give the patient.
- Consider environmental changes:
  - calming music,
  - avoid over-stimulation, e.g. television may worsen agitation,
  - objects may be misinterpreted, e.g a coat on the door may be perceived as a threatening man.
- Medication (Scottish Intercollegiate Guidelines Network, 1998):
  - all medication carries an increased risk of falls,
  - there is little good evidence as to the effectiveness for any drugs, although widely used,

Table 5.5. Drugs for behavioural disturbance

Antidepressants
- Co-morbid depression is common with behavioural problems
- Use if the patient has depressive or anxious symptoms
- Avoid TCAs – a risk of worsening confusion
- Consider a trial even in the absence of depressive symptoms

	Dose	Comments
Trazodone	50–250 mg	Sedative effect may help insomnia
Citalopram	20 mg	
Moclobemide	150–300 mg	

Neuroleptics
- Overall use shows 18% benefit over a placebo
- Only use if serious problems, in particular, psychotic symptoms, serious distress or danger
- Do not use in Lewy body dementia
- May hasten cognitive decline

Atypical neuroleptics

	Dose	Comments
Olanzapine	5 mg/day	Expensive (but using low
Risperidone	0.5–1 mg/day	doses); may be better tolerated than older drugs

Anticonvulsants
- Conflicting results from case reports and open trials

	Dose	Comment
Carbamazepine	100–800 mg/day	Reduces agitation and aggression Sedative
Sodium valproate	750–2500 mg	50% of a treatment-resistant group showed some response

Anticholinesterase inhibitors
- No trial evidence, but being used in clinical practice

(Adapted from Lanz and Marin, 1996)

- Medication (*continued*):
  - a high placebo effect,
  - if needed, use a low dose; review side-effects and efficacy regularly; short-term treatments,
  - avoid benzodiazepines because of dependence and worsening confusion.

Table 5.5 sets out possible drugs to consider.

In summary the management of agitated behaviour is:

- Consider non-drug causes and interventions.
- If the patient may be depressed or anxious, use an antidepressant:
  - trazodone, sedative,
  - citalopram, moclobemide.
- If the patient is psychotic or in severe distress try:
  - a low-dose neuroleptic, then
  - an antidepressant, then
  - carbamazepine.
- Keep under regular review.

Wandering

There is little research evidence in this field, but some simple measures have been shown to have some effect:

- Concealing door handles (behind a cloth).
- Putting a red 'STOP' sign in front of the exit door.

Sleep disturbance

- Avoid caffeine or stimulants.
- Manage night-time incontinence.
- Eliminate or restrict day-time napping.
- Increasing exercise or activity during the day.
- Avoid hypnotics if possible – consider trazodone if unavoidable.

Medico-legal issues

The GP may be called upon for an opinion as to the patient's capacity to manage their own affairs:

Testamentary capacity

To draw up and execute (sign) a will, individuals must be of *sound disposing mind*. They must:

- Understand they are giving their property to one or more 'objects of their regard'.
- Understand and recollect the extent of their property.
- Understand the nature and extent of the claims upon them (both those included and excluded) from the will.

The GP may be asked for an opinion at the time a will is drawn up, but more frequently may be asked to give a retrospective opinion following a contested will. In the second case clear, careful case records are, as ever, of great assistance.

Court of Protection

The Court of Protection manages the property and affairs of mentally disordered individuals (in England and Wales) who cannot manage for themselves. An application is made to the court by solicitors, social services or a patient's relatives. Such an application needs to be accompanied by a certificate of incapacity from either the patient's GP or a consultant psychiatrist.

Criteria for assessing incapacity are not identical with those for assessing the need for compulsory admission to hospital. The fact that a person is suffering from mental disorder is not of itself evidence of incapacity to manage their affairs.

The certificate requires the doctor to state the grounds on which their opinion of incapacity are based. What is required is not merely a diagnosis (although this may be included), but a simple statement giving clear evidence of incapacity which an intelligent lay person could understand, e.g. reference to defects of short-term memory, of spatial and temporal orientation or of reasoning ability.

Enduring power of attorney

Power of attorney is the mechanism whereby an individual empowers some-one else to act on their behalf, in a limited or unlimited capacity, in matters relating to finance and property. An ordinary power of attorney becomes invalid once the individual becomes incapable of managing their own affairs.

Enduring power of attorney is the mechanism which allows an individual, when well, to give power of attorney to someone else, to take effect either immediately or when they become mentally impaired. If the patient is unable to manage their affairs but still has the capacity to identify a trusted individual, enduring power of attorney can take effect immediately.

Use of the Mental Health Act

The Mental Health Act allows for the compulsory admission to hospital, and subsequent treatment, of patients with a mental disorder. The Act can be used, therefore, if necessary for the hospitalization and treatment of dementia and delirium. In that delirium has a physical cause, the most appropriate place for such patients if they need hospital treatment is a general hospital (although local arrangements may vary). The Mental Health Act can be used to admit patients to a general hospital although the use of the common law is often more apropriate. The case study below illustrates the use of the Mental Health Act in practice and the difficulties that arise.

CASE STUDY: JOAN

Dr Smith was called at 1.30 am by the Greenleigh Nursing Home about Joan, an 85-year-old patient who had been a resident of the nursing home for 9 months. Dr Smith had not met the patient before, but was informed by the night manager that she was suffering from dementia.

The reason for the telephone call was that Joan was screaming at fellow residents and staff saying, 'Keep away from me you f... Nazi, I know what you want.' She was hitting out at the staff who tried to guide her back to her chair, and was attempting to leave the nursing home and go out into the grounds. On one occasion she had been brought in from the garden.

Dr Smith visits Joan and finds an agitated woman who refuses to be examined and shouts, 'Go away you Nazi.' The nursing home record is not particularly informative, but does indicate that Joan is thought to be suffering from a vascular dementia and that she had carcinoma of the breast 10 years ago, successfully treated. Her current medication is tamoxifen 10 mg a day.

Dr Smith thinks that Joan may be hallucinating in that she keeps jerking her head and looking round as if responding to hallucinations. There is no previous history of psychiatric disorder other than her dementia.

After about an hour with Joan in which she tries to persuade her to take some diazepam or chlorpromazine, Dr Smith feels that Joan needs to be in hospital and calls the duty psychiatrist. The duty psychiatrist informs Dr Smith that it would not be appropriate for Joan to be admitted to the local mental hospital for what sounds like an acute confusional state. He suggests that Dr Smith tries to arrange for Joan's admission to the local geriatric unit. Dr Smith calls the geriatric registrar who says that they are happy to see Joan and an ambulance is called. Unfortunately, Joan refuses to get into the ambulance and the ambulance men refuse to take her to hospital against her will.

Dr Smith has now been up for 2.5 hours. Not knowing what to do next and aware that the nursing home staff are unable to cope, she manages together with the nursing staff to force a couple of tablets of diazepam into Joan's mouth, which eventually causes her to fall asleep.

Dr Smith visits the next morning and finds Joan to be drowsy, confused but no longer agitated. She is able to examine her and finds her to have a slight temperature. She discovers that she has been incontinent of urine for the past 2 days and makes a provisional diagnosis of a urinary tract infection and prescribes an antibiotic.

Dr Smith does not feel that the case was appropriately managed and rings her local psychogeriatrician to discuss what should happen in the future. Dr Smith is advised that the Mental Health Act could have been used to enable Joan to be transferred to hospital and be given treatment for her acute confusional state. She is also told that the ambulance team could have taken Joan into hospital under common law, in that Joan lacked capacity to make appropriate decisions about her care.

Although Dr Smith is now more certain of the legal position, she remains unclear about what would really be best for the patient in similar circumstances in the future.

Lessons from the case study

- Behavioural disturbance as the presentation of an acute confusional state in a lady with dementia.
- Medication is given under common law (which requires lack of capacity by the patient, necessity and a judgement of the patient's best interests).
- The Mental Health Act could have been used to admit the patient to the general hospital.

The Mental Health Act can also be used for patients requiring guardianship. This provision of the Act allows a 'guardian' (a relative or the local authority) to require the patient to live in a certain place, e.g. a nursing home, and to allow access to health and care staff.

National Assistance Act

The National Assistance Act (section 47) allows a magistrate to order the removal to a suitable place of a person suffering from:

- Grave chronic disease, or being aged, infirm, incapacitated and living in unsanitary conditions.
- Unable to care for themselves.

Applications are usually made by a public health consultant.

When to refer

If considering referral it is helpful for the specialist services if there has been a recent cardiovascular and neurological examination together with the physical investigations on page 125.

WHEN TO REFER

- Early diagnosis of a dementing illness to ensure:
  - appropriate differential diagnosis,
  - treatment where available, e.g. use of anticholinesterase inhibitors for mild-to-moderate Alzheimer's disease,
  - appropriate planning by the patient and relatives.
- Access to specialist services:
  - respite care,
  - home nursing.
- Dementia associated with agitated or psychotic features.
- Atypical dementia:
  - early onset,
  - rapid progression.

What to expect from secondary care

Assessment and advice

Patients with possible dementia should be assessed, and an appropriate diagnosis made. A plan for future care should be agreed with the patient, their carers, primary care and social services.

Memory clinic

Many areas will have set up a specialist memory clinic for the assessment of patients with early dementia, and the consideration of treatment with drugs for Alzheimer's disease.

DRUGS FOR ALZHEIMER'S DISEASE

Anticholinesterase inhibitors – Donepezil, Rivastigmine, Galantamine – act by preventing the breakdown of acetylcholine at nerve endings.

Benefit
- Approximately 50% of patients with mild/moderate dementia (mini mental state examination 10–26) show some cognitive improvement occurring between 12 and 18 weeks.
- Some reports of improved functioning.
- Benefit lasts 9–12 months.

Side-effects
- Well tolerated.
- Some gastrointestinal disturbance.
- Anticholinergic effects.

Current recommendation
Prescribed by specialists with clear monitoring of response.

The NICE Guidance (2001) on drugs for Alzheimer's disease recommend the use of drugs when:

- Diagnosis of Alzheimer's disease is made in a specialist clinic.
- The mini mental state examination score is 12 or above.
- A carer can ensure compliance.
- Assessment at 2 to 4 months to determine the benefit.
- Six-monthly reviews.
- Stop the drug when the mini mental state examination score is below 12.

Gingo biloba (currently classified in the UK as a foodstuff and available without restriction) has been shown to improve cognitive function and is well tolerated (Warner and Butler, 2001).

Respite care
Repite care may be provided by health services or by social services.

Support and co-ordination of care
Support and co-ordination of care for patients with moderate-to-severe disorder and of those with challenging behaviours.

Acute confusional state (delirium)
An acute confusional state is a syndrome characterized by:

- Acute onset (a few hours).
- Moderately brief duration (days).
- Disorientation in time and place.
- Global cognitive impairment.
- Fluctuating course.

It is associated with behavioural, perceptual and emotional disturbances. Acute confusional states are caused by a range of medical conditions, drugs and alcohol.

The management of acute confusional states has two components:

- Identification and treatment of the underlying cause.
- Symptomatic management of symptoms – if drug treatment is unavoidable, use of the medication drawn from Table 5.5 (page 130) may be appropriate.

REFERENCES

Eccles, Clarke J, Livingston M *et al.* (1998). North of England evidence based guidelines development project: guideline for the primary care management of dementia. *British Medical Journal* **317**:802–7.

Folstein MF, Folstein SE, McHuch PR (1975). Mini mental state. A practical method for grading the cognitive state of patients for the clinician. *Journal of Psychiatric Research* **12**:189–98.

Frank P (1998). Dementia workup. *Canadian Family Physician* **44:**1489–95.

Lantz MS, Marin D (1996). Pharmacologic treatment of agitation in dementia: a comprehensive review. *Journal of Geriatric Psychiatry and Neurology* **9:**107–19.

National Institute for Clinical Excellence (2001). *Guidance on the use of donepezil, rivastigmine and galantamine for the treatment of Alzheimer's disease.* NICE, London.

Scottish Intercollegiate Guidelines Network (1998). Twenty-two interventions in the management of behavioural and psychological aspects of dementia. www.sho.scot.nhs.uk/sign.

Siu AL (1991). Screening for dementia and investigating its causes. *Annals of Internal Medicine* **115:**112–32.

Small GW, Rabins PV, Barry PP *et al.* (1997). Diagnosis and treatment of Alzheimer's disease and related disorders. Consensus statement of the American Association for Geriatric Psychiatry, The Alzheimer's Association and the American Geriatric Society. *Journal of the American Medical Association* **278:**1363–71.

Stewart JT (1991). Managing the care of patients with dementia. *Postgraduate Medicine* **90:**45–9.

Streiner D, Geddes J (1998). Some useful concepts and terms used in articles about diagnosis. *Evidence Based Mental Health* **1:**6–7.

Walstra GJM, Teunisse S, van Gool WA *et al.* (1997). Reversible dementia in elderly patients referred to a memory clinic. *Journal of Neurology* **224:**17–22.

Warner J, Butler R (2001). Alzheimer's Disease in *Clinical Evidence.* Issue 4. BMJ Publishing Group, London.

Wind AW, Schellevis FG, Van Staveren G, Scholten R, Jonker C, Van Eijk J (1997). Limitations of the mini mental state examination in diagnosing dementia in general practice. *International Journal of Geriatric Psychiatry* **12:**101–8.

FURTHER READING

Jacoby R, Oppenheimer C (1991). *Psychiatry in the Elderly.* OUP Oxford.

WEBSITES

Age Info

www.cpa.org.uk/ageinfo/ageinfo.html

Provides information for anyone concerned with older people.

The Alzheimer Page
www.biostat.wustl.edu/alzheimer
US site with general information about Alzheimer's disease.

SELF-HELP

Age Concern
Astral House, 1268 London Road, Norbury, London SW16 4ER
Tel: 202 8679 8000 (England)
    0131 220 3345 (Scotland)
    01222 371566 (Wales)
    01232 245729 (Ireland)
Websites: www.ace.org.uk
    www.ace.org.uk/cymru/default.htm (Wales)

Help the Aged
St James Walk, London EC1R 0BE
Tel: 020 7253 0253
    0800 650065 (freephone)

Alzheimer's Disease Society
Gordon House, 10 Greencoat Place, London SW10 1PH
Tel: 020 7306 0606
    0845 300 0336 (helpline)
Website: www.alzheimers.org.uk

Carers National Association
20–25 Glasshouse Yard, London EC1A HJS
Tel: 020 7490 8818

Counsel and Care
Twyman House, 16 Bonny Street, London NW1 9PG
Tel: 020 7485 1566
Advice and help for older people.

Tripscope
Tel: 0345 585641
Nationwide travel and transport information and advice service for disabled and elderly people.

Seniorline (Help the Aged)
Freephone: 0800 289404
Provides help and advice for elderly people.

Compassionate Friends
53 North Street, Bristol BS3 1EN
Tel: 01272 539639
Provides help for relatives of patients with dementia.

National Association of Widows
54–57 Alison Street, Digbeth, Birmingham B5 5TH
Tel: 0121 643 8348

chapter 6

The patient with somatic symptoms

IN THIS CHAPTER

- How to identify medically unexplained (somatic) symptoms.
- Primary care management of:
  - acute somatic symptoms,
  - chronic somatic symptoms,
- Heartsink and hateful patients.

INTRODUCTION

Medically unexplained physical symptoms are common in both primary and secondary care. Somatization describes the presentation of psychological distress as physical symptoms. Somatizing patients are high utilizers of medical care and can be frustrating patients to care for.

EPIDEMIOLOGY

Medically unexplained (somatic) symptoms are common in primary care (Table 6.1) and are usually associated with depression, anxiety, or concurrent substance misuse. Chronic somatic symptoms are less common, but result in a significant workload. In a general practice sample from Southampton of consecutive attenders, 19% were thought by their GP to have clinically signif-

Table 6.1. Epidemiology of somatization

- Approximately 70% of patients with an emotional disorder present in primary care with a somatic complaint
- 20% of new presentations of illness in primary care are medically unexplained symptoms
- Acute somatic symptoms are associated with
  - depression
  - anxiety
  - substance misuse
- 1 in 5 surgery attenders have chronic somatic symptoms (duration 2 years plus)

icant medically unexplained symptoms of at least 3 months' duration. A larger proportion (35%) were picked up on screening as having a minimum of four in men, or six in women, unexplained medical symptoms (Peveler *et al.*, 1997).

In a US study of 1000 patients from four primary care sites, 8% were found to have three or more medically unexplained, currently bothersome symptoms of at least 2 years' duration. These patients had equivalent impairment in their quality of life and social disability as patients with mood and anxiety disorders (Kroenke *et al.*, 1998).

Recognition and diagnosis

The first task of the GP when presented with a patient with physical symptoms is to determine whether or not there is a medical cause. This task is made more difficult because the presence of physical symptoms, irrespective of aetiology, is associated with increased social and psychiatric morbidity. In adults, symptoms that commonly turn out to be medically unexplained include chest, back or abdominal pain, tiredness, dizziness, headache, ankle swelling, shortness of breath, insomnia and numbness. Physical symptoms such as these prompt almost half of all primary care consultations, but are shown to have an organic origin in only about 10–15% of patients followed up for 1 year (Drugs and Therapeutics Bulletin, 2001).

There are pointers to making a positive diagnosis of medically unexplained symptoms rather than solely relying on a diagnosis of exclusion:

POINTERS FOR DIAGNOSIS OF MEDICALLY UNEXPLAINED SYMPTOMS

- Symptom description: vague, inconsistent, fluctuating.
- Level of concern is disproportionate to symptoms.
- Frequent attenders.
- Much doctoring, little curing.
- Changes of doctor due to dissatisfaction.
- Denial of possible psychological role in symptoms.
- Associated psychiatric illness.

(Kaplan *et al.*, 1988)

Acute somatic symptoms are usually associated with another psychiatric disorder:

- If low mood, consider depression.
- If seeking pain relief, consider drug misuse.
- If prominent anxiety symptoms, consider anxiety disorder.
- If strange beliefs about symptoms, consider acute psychosis.

The primary health care version of ICD-10 (ICD-10 PHC) has unexplained somatic complaints as a diagnostic term.

UNEXPLAINED SOMATIC COMPLAINTS – ICD-10 PHC

- Many physical symptoms without medical explanation (proper history and physical examinations are necessary to determine this).
- May be overly concerned about medical illness.
- Symptoms of depression and anxiety are common.
- Frequent medical visits and negative investigations.

Chronic somatic symptoms may be a feature of somatization disorder or hypochondriasis.

ICD-10 DIAGNOSTIC FEATURES OF SOMATIZATION DISORDER

- At least 2 years of multiple and variable physical symptoms for which no adequate physical explanation has been found.
- Persistent refusal to accept the advice or reassurance of several doctors that there is no physical explanation for the symptoms.
- Some degree of impairment of social and family functioning.

Hypochondriasis differs from somatization in that the focus is fear of an underlying disease or illness, rather than a focus on individual symptoms.

MANAGEMENT IN PRIMARY CARE

Gask *et al.* (1989) have developed a training course to teach GPs the skills to manage somatic symptoms. The technique taught (reattribution) has three stages:

- *Ensuring the patient feels understood* by taking a full symptoms history, responding to mood cues, asking about family and social factors, exploring health beliefs and carrying out a brief, focussed physical examination.
- *Changing the agenda* from a discussion of physical symptoms to psychological symptoms.
- *Making the link* between the physical and psychological symptoms.

GPs trained in these techniques:

- Reduce symptom levels in patients.
- Reduce specialist referrals.
- No extra burden on primary care (Morris *et al.*, 1998).

Ensuring the patient feels understood

Time must be given for the patient to tell the doctor their symptoms and be appropriately questioned and examined.

Changing the agenda

Move from discussion of physical symptoms to psychological symptoms:

'Have you noticed any other problems?'
'Have you been feeling down, sad or depressed lately?' (Depression.)
'Have you lost interest in activities you previously enjoyed?' (Depression.)
'Have you been feeling tense, or anxious, or worrying a lot?' (Anxiety.)
'In the past few weeks how much alcohol would you drink per day and how many times a week would you drink alcohol?' (Alcohol use.)

Making the link

How to help the patient accept a non-medical explanation for their symptoms.

Acknowledge that symptoms are real

It is important to acknowledge that symptoms are real and not imagined. The fact that no physical cause can be found does not mean there is nothing wrong or that there are no symptoms.

'Just because no physical cause can be found does not mean that there is nothing wrong with you or that you have no symptoms. There is something causing this and I can see that it is worrying you a great deal; but it is not a serious medical problem. Perhaps it might be linked to the other problems you have told me about and the worries you have at the moment. What do you think?'

Stress and tension can lead to physical symptoms
An explanation for patients is set out below.

How stress and tension lead to physical problems

- First, worry and tension can cause you to tighten up your muscles. When this lasts for some time these muscles can become painful (remember what it was like the last time you carried heavy bags for a long time – your arms will have been hurting). When this happens to the muscles at the back of the neck, it leads to headache. When muscles around the bowel contract it leads to stomach pains.
- Second, when you get tense and anxious this causes a substance called adrenalin to be released into your body. This can be very helpful in making you more alert and prepared to deal with problems, but unfortunately it can cause many physical symptoms, e.g. racing heart.
- Third, breathing too quickly and/or deeply (also known as hyperventiliation) decreases levels of carbon dioxide. Symptoms include dizziness, light-headedness, breathlessness, feelings of unreality, pounding heart, tingling sensations and so on.
- Fourth, if you are feeling down or fed up, you are much more likely to focus on your bodily sensations and worry about them than when you are feeling cheerful. If you have played sport remember the difference between how much an injury hurt when you were on the losing side compared to when you were winning!
- Finally, we focus in and worry about some symptoms more than others. If a member of your family or a friend has had a life-threatening illness which began with the symptoms that you are experiencing now, you will tend to worry more about this.

(Adapted from WHO Guide to Mental Health in Primary Care (2000)

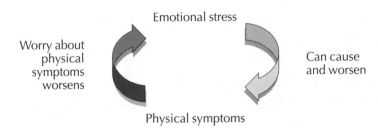

Emotional stress

Worry about physical symptoms worsens

Can cause and worsen

Physical symptoms

Figure 6.1. Relationship between stress and physical symptoms.

In simple terms, a vicious circle can be set up (Figure 6.1).

The management of acute somatic symptoms is simpler than when the symptoms have become chronic. When working with chronic somatizing patients, time and patience is needed. Such patients are often very sensitive to being dismissed as 'there is nothing wrong with you'. A suggestion that the patient might benefit from a psychiatric referral is often seen as rejection. The principles of changing the agenda and making the link between physical symptoms and psychological problems applies with chronic just as with acute somatic symptoms. However, a slower pace is needed and goals should be more limited. Goldberg *et al.* (1992) set out key ideas for the management of acute and chronic somatization in primary care (Tables 6.2 and 6.3).

Table 6.2. Management of acute somatic symptoms

Ensuring the patient feels understood
- Why has the patient consulted?
  - ?symptom relief
  - ?diagnostic test and reassurance
- Identification of the relevant stressors including fear of illness
- Brief focussed physical evaluation to reassure the patient that a medical problem is not being overlooked

Changing the agenda
Consider depression, alcohol, substance misuse

Continued on page 150

Table 6.2 (*continued*)

Making the link
- Reassurance that there is no physical disease requiring medical treatment
- An explanation linking stress and distress to the physical symptoms

Further management
Appropriate management of the underlying stressors or depressive disorder:
- Consider a problem-solving approach
- Encourage exercise and enjoyable activities
- Give a reducing stress handout (Figure 6.2)

Table 6.3. Management of chronic somatic symptoms

- Reassurance that nothing is wrong does not help
- The patient wants the physician to agree that they are sick. The physician should avoid challenging the patient, agree there is a problem, and show a willingness to help identify it. The physician should acknowledge the patient's plight
- Little is to be gained by a premature explanation that the symptoms are emotional. Such an explanation must be presented in such a way that the patient does not experience it as rejection. Patients will often say, 'I feel depressed because of my symptoms.'
- The emphasis of treatment should be on function, not symptoms. 'Can we try and work together on helping you lead as active a life as possible despite these symptoms?'
- Regular scheduled appointments are required so that the patient does not have to manifest symptoms to seek help. 'Perhaps we could meet regularly to check up on how you are rather than only seeing you when things are very bad.'
- The physician should reinforce non-illness behaviours and communication
- Diagnostic tests should be limited. Some focussed examination can be helpful, with reliance more on signs than symptoms

Reducing stress

Accepting personal responsibility for your life ...

1 Work no more than 10 hours daily.
2 Have at least half an hour for each meal ... and don't work while eating!
3 Have at least one and a half days per week free from work.
4 Cultivate a habit of listening to relaxing music ... or even better – learn to PLAY it!
5 Learn a form of relaxation/meditation and try to give some time to this regularly.
6 Walk and talk at a slower pace ... WATCH YOURSELF!
7 Try to take some regular, mild exercise (swimming, walking, cycling, badminton)
8 Examine your eating habits and diet (reduce caffeine, sugar, salt, and saturated fats).
9 Cultivate a hobby that is ceative rather than competitive.
10 If emotional or sexual relationships are upsetting, seek advice.
11 If unhappy at work ... take stock.
12 Concentrate on the PRESENT, avoiding the tendency to dwell on the past or future uncertainties.
13 Do not accept or set yourself unrealistic deadlines or standards.
14 Give yourself 'permission' to pamper yourself ... treat yourself as you would treat a good friend. Ease up on yourself, focussing more on your good points and avoiding any tendency to dwell on self-criticism.

Some additional points to remember:

Slow down
Pace your activities
Cut down on tea, coffee, cigarettes, alcohol
Notice early signs of tension ... and STOP!
Remember that stress symptoms cannot harm you
Do one thing at a time – not several things at once
Establish a balance of work vs play
Cut down on the 'negatives' – aimed at self or others
Have breaks and stops – take 'time out' more often
Look at realistic change – plan it – then do it!

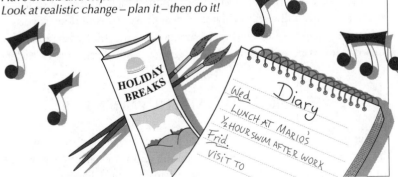

Figure 6.2. Reducing stress handout.

Antidepressants can be useful in the treatment of patients with medically unexplained symptoms, such as fatigue, poor sleep and pain, whether or not depression is present. Before starting an antidepressant, it is important to explain to the patient that the drug is not being used primarily to treat depression, but to help symptoms. (Tricyclic antidepressants are licenced only for the treatment of depression.) Treatment should start at a low dose of the drug and be increased gradually (usually at weekly intervals according to the response). Benefit is usually seen within 1–7 days of starting treatment (i.e. before any antidepressant effect would be expected to occur) (Drugs and Therapeutics Bulletin, 2001).

Frequent attenders

Somatizing patients are frequent attenders in primary care. Frequent attenders to primary care have been identified as falling into five categories:

- Patients with entirely physical illnesses.
- Patients with clear psychiatric illnesses.
- Patients in acute crisis.
- Chronically somatizing patients.
- Patients with multiple problems.

The reason for presentation in all groups is usually for physical illnesses or physical symptoms. The management of the frequent attender will clearly depend on the cause. A recognition of frequent attendance should alert the doctor to possible psychiatric disorder.

If depressive disorders are recognized amongst high utilizers of service care and treated, this will result in significant improvements in depressive symptomatology, quality of life and social functioning, together with reduced days missed from work and reduced health-service costs (Katzelnick *et al.*, 1997).

THE HEARTSINK AND HATEFUL PATIENT

Chronic somatizers can be frustrating patients to care for. Acknowledging the fact that some patients can be irritating and unrewarding can be helpful in avoiding personal burnout. 'Heartsink survival' has been suggested as comprising the following coping strategies:

Heartsink survival

- Share difficulties with a colleague.
- Set clear boundaries:
  - how often to see the patient,
  - how long,
  - what will I do?
- Set goals for what you want to achieve with the patient, e.g.:
  - decrease hospital referrals,
  - increase patient activities.
- Accept powerlessness and not be drawn into the patient's demands for a cure.

(Mathers *et al.*, 1995)

Groves (1978) identifies 'hateful patients', i.e. 'those whom most physicians dread'. These include dependent clingers, entitled demanders and manipulative help-rejecters.

Dependent clingers

Patients who have a bottomless need for care and see their physician as inexhaustible. Their initial gratitude changes to resentment.

Management of these patients includes:

- Clear limits to appointments.
- Follow-up appointments offered with a request not to come earlier except for emergencies.
- Informing the patient that there is a limit to your time and stamina.

Entitled demanders

As with clingers, these patients have a profound need for care, but use hostility to gain more attention. They often demand more investigations, opinions and treatment.

Management of these patients includes:

- Acknowledging the patient's needs.
- Repeating that such needs should be met by the provision of first-rate medical care rather than by the specific demands requested.

Manipulative help-rejecters

Like clingers and demanders, such patients demand attention and time, but are clear that no treatment will help: 'Yes ... but-ers'.

Management of these patients includes:

- Acknowledging the difficulties of treatment.
- Focussing on patient-set goals – function rather than symptoms.

It can be seen how chronic somatizers could fall into these categories. Recognition of the difficulties such patients present can be helpful both for the doctor and patient.

WHEN TO REFER

The skill in managing somatizing patients is to avoid medical and surgical referrals together with attendant investigations. Psychiatric referral can be a difficult task in itself as many patients will refuse to attend. Psychiatric referral should be considered if:

- The patient would like help to manage psychosocial stressors underpinning the somatization.
- The patient has an associated psychiatric disorder, e.g. depression or substance misuse, which has not responded to simple treatment measures.
- The GP needs help in restricting multiple hospital referrals and/or investigations. (Note, the patient may be unwilling to attend.)

Role of secondary care

Secondary care has a limited role in the treatment of somatization. Specialist psychological help may assist the GP in the management of the most difficult patients, particularly those who are using a lot of secondary services. It can, however, be very difficult both to persuade the patient to attend for an initial assessment or to engage them in a psychological treatment.

Cognitive behaviour therapy is the treatment of choice for medically unexplained symptoms. The treatment encourages self-help techniques, such as relaxation and self-management of stress and anxiety. The patient is encouraged to keep a diary of symptoms, thoughts and evidence for and against there being a serious cause for their symptoms. Cognitive behaviour therapy discourages maintaining factors, such as repeated body checking, and challenges the patient's negative or false beliefs about symptoms.

REFERENCES

Drugs and Therapeutics Bulletin (2001). What to do about medically unexplained symptoms. *Drugs and Therapeutics Bulletin* **39**:5–7.

Gask L, Goldberg D, Porter R, Creed F (1989). The treatment of somatisation: evaluation of a teaching package with general practice trainees. *Journal of Psychosomatic Research* **33**:697–703.

Goldberg RJ, Hovack DH, Gask L (1992). The recognition and management of somatisation. *Psychosomatics* **33**:55–61.

Groves JE (1978). Taking care of the hateful patient. *New England Journal of Medicine* **198**:883–7.

Kaplan C, Lipkin M, Gordon GH (1988). Somatization in primary care. *Journal of General International Medicine* **3**:177–89.

Katzelnick DJ, Kobak, Greist J, Jefferson JW, Henky HJ (1997). Effects of primary care treatment of depression on service use by patients with high medical expenditures. *Psychiatric Services* **48**:59–64.

Kroenke K, Spitler RL, DeGruif V, Hahn SR, Linzer M, Williams J, Brody D, Davies M (1998). Multi-somataform disorder: An alternative to undifferentiated somataform disorders for the somatising patient in primary care. *Archives of General Psychiatry* **55**:352–8.

Mathers N, Jones N, Hanney D (1995). Heartsink patients: A study of their general practitioners. *British Journal of General Practice* **45**:293–6.

Morriss R, Gask L, Ronalds C, Downs-Grainger E, Thompson H, Leese B, Goldberg D (1998). Cost effectiveness of a new treatment for somatized mental disorder taught to GPs. *Family Practice* **15:**119–24.

Peveler R, Kilkenny L, Kinmouth A (1997). Medically unexplained physical symptoms in primary care. *Journal of Psychosomatic Research* **42:**245–52.

WHO Guide to Mental Health in Primary Care (2000). Royal Society of Medicine Press, London.

chapter 7

The patient with insomnia

IN THIS CHAPTER

- Checklist of medical and psychological causes of insomnia.
- Non-drug interventions for insomnia:
  - sleep hygiene,
  - stimulus control,
  - sleep restriction.
- Which drug treatments to consider and when.

INTRODUCTION

Advising those with sleep problems on what to do is an activity common in both general practice and everyday life. Much of such advice is common sense, some evidence based and some folklore. There are a range of effective drug and non-drug interventions for insomnia. This chapter will set out a systematic approach to the management of sleep problems in primary care.

Insomnia is the perception, or complaint, of inadequate or poor-quality sleep because of one or more of the following:

- Difficulty falling asleep.
- Waking up frequently during the night with difficulty returning to sleep.
- Waking too early in the morning.
- Unrefreshing sleep.

Insomnia is *not* defined by the number of hours asleep, or how long it takes to fall asleep. Insomnia can be temporary or chronic. Temporary insomnia, e.g. related to jetlag, environmental disturbance, hyperarousal (worry or pain) or a bereavement, needs to be distinguished from more persistent symptoms.

EPIDEMIOLOGY

Insomnia is a symptom and not a diagnosis. Few surveys either in community or primary care samples have focussed on insomnia itself, information about sleep having been collected as part of a wider survey. Figures about the prevalence of insomnia often, therefore, focus on different criteria and can mean very different things (Table 7.1).

Studies from the community and primary care indicate that insomnia results in a considerable economic burden, resulting in reduced productivity, increased absenteeism, increased accidents, and increased use of general medical resources (Simon and Von Korff, 1997). There is evidence that insomnia causes disability in its own right, in addition to its association with other conditions, such as depression and harmful use of alcohol.

Table 7.1. Epidemiology of sleep problems

- Community prevalence (UK): self report sleep problem 25%
- Primary care prevalence (USA): 2 hours + to fall asleep 10%
- Primary care prevalence (UK): self report sleep difficulties 60%
- Level of disability is similar to that of anxiety disorders (3–4 disability days a month)
- Insomnia is as powerful a predictor of early death as obesity

Is insomnia more frequent in the elderly?

The answer is probably 'yes', but this needs to be qualified. Older people are more often troubled by night-time awakenings rather than difficulty getting off to sleep – clearly there may be physical causes for this. There is also an increased frequency of daytime napping. In a Nottingham primary care sample of 1042 patients, aged 65 and over, just over 20% reported severely disrupted sleep, with a new incident rate of about 3% (Morgan and Clarke, 1997). Chronic sleep disturbance in the elderly is associated with being female, depressed, living alone, taking psychotropic medication and activity limitation.

Despite the frequency of the symptom and the desire by patients for help, most patients do not consult their doctor about the insomnia with a mutual, 'Don't ask, don't tell', policy in force.

CAUSES OF INSOMNIA

In general practice samples, there are three major conditions associated with insomnia: depression, substance abuse and physical illness (Table 7.2).

Table 7.2. Causes of insomnia in primary care

Depression
- Approximately 30% of patients with insomnia have a moderate depressive disorder
- Insomnia is an important symptom in depressive disorders
- Untreated insomnia leads to an increased incidence of depression

Substance abuse
Substances to consider include:
- Alcohol
- Hypnotics
- Caffeine
- Illicit drugs

Physical illness
- Painful illnesses
- Chronic medical illnesses
- Nocturnal asthma
- Movement disorders

People also wake up because of environmental factors, e.g. noise and temperature. In a sample from Dorset primary care, 40% of people who woke up gave the reason as 'going to the toilet'.

MANAGEMENT IN PRIMARY CARE

✓ Psychological causes.
✓ Physical causes.
✓ Lifestyle causes.
✓ Sleep hygiene.
✓ Stimulus control.
✓ Sleep restriction.
✓ Drug treatments.

The symptom of insomnia is a perception combining inadequate time asleep, inadequate quality of sleep and an unacceptable sleep pattern. Assessment includes determining the number of hours the patient is asleep and an assessment of the impact of the insomnia on daytime functioning. It can be helpful for patients to keep a sleep diary over two weeks recording: bedtime, time of waking, meals, exercise, medication and alcohol together with the duration and quality of sleep.

The management of insomnia can be set out as a series of stages:

Diagnosis: is there a psychological cause?

Depressive disorder
Ask about other depressive and anxious symptoms:

'Sleep problems are common during times of stress. Have you been feeling down or depressed recently? Have you lost interest in activities you previously enjoyed? Have you been feeling tense of anxious or worrying about minor matters?'

- Treat the underlying disorder with an antidepressant.
- Consider a sedative antidepressant, e.g. amitriptyline, trazodone, mirtazapine.

Substance misuse

- Ask about alcohol, hypnotics and non-prescribed drugs

'Sometimes lifestyle interferes with sleep – shall we look at some things which might be affecting your sleep? What about alcohol? In the last few weeks how much alcohol would you drink per day? How many times a week? How about tea or coffee, soft drinks? Any non-prescribed pills?'

- Consider caffeine use, caffeine has a half-life of 5 hours. Table 7.3 lists common sources of caffeine.

Table 7.3 Common sources of caffeine

Product		Caffeine content (mg) Range	Mean
Instant coffee	1 cup (150 ml)	40–180	59
Percolated coffee	1 cup (150 ml)	64–124	83
Decaffeinated coffee	1 cup (150 ml)	2–5	3
Tea (content increases with brewing)	1 cup (150 ml)	8–91	27
Cocoa: S. American	1 cup (150 ml)		42
African	1 cup (150 ml)		6
Cola drinks	12 oz can	40–60	45
Milk chocolate bar	60 mg		40
Many over-the-counter drugs have a high caffeine content			

(Stradling, 1993)

Dementia

This is associated with a breakdown in the circadian rhythm.

Diagnosis: is there a physical cause?

If the patient presents with pain, identify and treat the cause of the pain. Give appropriate analgesia.

In the event of a medical disorder, treat appropriately.

MEDICAL CAUSES OF INSOMNIA

- Breathlessness: nocturnal asthma, paroxysmal nocturnal dyspnoea.
- Nocturia: prostatic disease, infections, renal disease.
- Endocrine disorders: diabetes with thirst, hyperthyroidism.
- Prescribed drugs: several drugs both during therapy and withdrawal (see below).
- Sleep apnoea: 'Has anyone complained about your snoring?'

COMMON PRESCRIPTION DRUGS KNOWN TO CAUSE INSOMNIA

Antihypertensives
Clonidine
Betablockers
Methyldopa

Anticholinergics

Hormones
Oral contraceptives
Thyroid preparations
Cortisone
Progesterone

Sympathomimetic amines
Bronchodilators
Xanthine derivatives
Theophylline
Decongestants
Phenylpropanolamine
Pseudoephedrine

Antineoplastics

Miscellaneous
Phenytoin
Nicotine
Levodopa
Quinidine
Caffeine (over-the-counter products)

(Kupfer and Reynolds, 1997)

Is there a lifestyle cause?

Many patients do not sleep well because of taking part in activities that interfere with the maintenance of good-quality sleep. Patients should be advised to alter habits that result in poor sleep hygiene.

Sleep hygiene is based on a series of common-sense principles. There is evidence that patients with insomnia benefit from such an intervention. A word of caution, however:

'Many mental health professionals hand their patients little pamphlets filled with "sleep hygiene rules". This is no more effective, in my experience, than handing a neurotic patient a list of "rules for healthy emotional living". The therapist should keep the sleep hygiene rules in his or her own mind and use them judiciously when discussing the particular sleep problem with a patient. I have rarely found a patient who can benefit from more than three or four individually tailored rules at any given time.' (Hauri, 1979)

Table 7.4 (overleaf) gives sleep hygiene rules.

Other psychological interventions to treat insomnia

If there is no psychological, physical or lifestyle cause for the insomnia and not sleeping is a persistent problem, three simple psychological interventions can be tried: stimulus control, sleep restriction or relaxation (Morin *et al.*, 1994; Murtagh and Greenwood, 1995).

Table 7.4. Sleep hygiene rules

Reduce time in bed
- Do not spend time awake in bed (get up read/listen to music)
- Avoid daytime naps (in bed or elsewhere)

Avoid caffeine, alcohol and nicotine
- Low doses of alcohol promote sleep, but as alcohol is metabolized sleep becomes disturbed
- Avoid caffeine from the afternoon onwards

Exercise in the late afternoon or early evening
- Exercise is helpful early in the day, but leads to over-arousal in the evening

Regular bedtime
- Go to bed at the same time
- Get up at a pre-set time whatever sleep is obtained

Eliminate the bedroom clock
- Once the alarm is set, hide the clock away and do not keep looking at it

Avoid stimulating/upsetting activity before sleep
- Do not do work in the late evening
- Avoid arguments in the evening
- Set a worry time for earlier in the day

Get the environment right
- Comfortable bed
- Bedroom neither too hot or cold
- Quiet (consider ear plugs)
- Blackout light

Eat a light bedtime snack
- Do not eat a main meal late in the evening
- Milky drinks contain tryptophan which may help

Stimulus control

Stimulus control is a set of instructions designed to reduce sleep incompatible behaviours and to develop a consistent sleep-wake cycle. Combining the results of about 20 studies indicates that the time taken to fall asleep and the time awake after falling asleep is reduced by half. The rationale underpinning the treatment is that the bedroom has become associated with a frustrated desire to sleep and performance anxiety has set in about sleep. Stimulus control acts to change this.

STIMULUS CONTROL INSTRUCTIONS

1 Use your bedroom only for sleep and sex. Do not read, watch television or eat in bed, and do not use the bedroom for work.
2 Go to bed only when you are sleepy.
3 If you are in bed for more than about 15 minutes without falling asleep, you should get up and try again later:
  – go to another room and stay up as long as you wish and engage in an undemanding activity, e.g. reading, watching TV,
  – return to your bedroom only when you are sleepy,
  – the goal is to associate your bed with falling asleep quickly.
4 Repeat step (3) as necessary. Once your mind has accepted the association of the bedroom with sleep, repeats will be less necessary.
5 Set your alarm and get up at the same time every morning regardless of the amount of sleep you have had during the night.
6 Do not nap during the day.

Sleep restriction

Sleep restriction therapy consists of curtailing the amount of time in bed to the actual amount of sleep. It is about as effective as stimulus control, but has been evaluated in fewer studies. It is often most helpful for older patients who may over-estimate their need for sleep. The technique is used for patients who spend considerable time in bed awake.

The patient is instructed to restrict their time in bed only to the number of hours that they sleep. Thus if the patient is only sleeping 4 hours a night, they should be told to only go to bed for 4 hours. Patients may initially feel tired during the day as they often under estimate the amount of time they are sleeping. As with the stimulus control method, patients will gradually learn to associate going to bed with going to sleep rather than with lying awake anxiously. Patients keep a sleep/wake diary. The allowable time in bed is increased by 15–20 minutes for each week when sleep time is over 90% of the time in bed. The allowable time is reduced by the same amount if sleep time is under 80% of total time in bed. Adjustments are made periodically until an adequate sleep-wake cycle is achieved.

SLEEP RESTRICTION

- Stay in bed for only the hours you sleep, e.g. if only 4 hours go to bed at 1.00 am and get up at 5.00 am.
- Keep a sleep diary and record the amount of time asleep.
- If you are asleep more than 90% of the time in bed – over a week – spend an extra 15 minutes in bed.
- If you are asleep less than 80% of the time in bed – over a week – spend 15 minutes less in bed.
- Do not sleep during the day.

Relaxation

Several studies using different relaxation techniques have shown some benefit from relaxation. Relaxation classes may be available within primary care, or patients can be directed to the self-help tapes and books which are readily available.

Consider drug treatments

There are a range of effective drugs to assist patients with insomnia. Many of these drugs also carry the risk of dependence and tolerance. However, as Table 7.5 shows, hypnotics are regularly prescribed in England. The table does not include the use of sedative antidepressant drugs which are widely used as an aid to sleep.

Table 7.5 Prescriptions for hypnotic drugs (England, 1997)	
Temazepam	5 252 000
Nitrazepam	2 425 000
Zopiclone	1 679 000
Chlormethiazole	280 000
Lormetazepam	248 000
Chloral hydrate	246 000
Loprazolam	215 000
Zolpidem	209 000

Drugs really only have a role in temporary insomnia. Temporary insomnia may be associated with daytime sleepiness, irritability, impaired concentration with the risk of accidents at work, home or on the road, hence a brief course of medication may be appropriate. In chronic insomnia, drugs are easy to start, initially effective, but then tolerance develops and dependence makes them difficult to stop.

Benzodiazepines
Benzodiazepines are widely used for the treatment of insomnia in general practice, reflecting the fact they are tried, tested and relatively inexpensive. The advice in the BNF about the use of benzodiazepines to treat insomnia is that they should be used 'only when it is severe, disabling or subjecting the individual to extreme distress'. The risks of dependence are well known and such drugs should only be given in short courses of 1–2 weeks at a time. Benzodiazepines with a short half-life, such as temazepam and oxazepam (both 8 hours), are to be preferred over drugs with a longer half-life, such as nitrazepam (30 hours) and diazepam (32 hours). Two schools of thought exist, either to use the drugs on an as-required basis to help limit dependence, or to use in a brief prescribed course because of the risk of rebound insomnia following use over even one night.

Benzodiazepines are popular with patients – over 70% of patients who have been prescribed a benzodiazepine over the pervious year as a hypnotic would take the medication again for the same purpose.

Sedative antidepressants

Low doses of sedative antidepressants, such as amitriptyline and dothiepin, can be used as an inexpensive hypnotic. Both these drugs have anticholinergic side-effects, however, which may limit their use even in low doses. Trazodone, a sedative serotonin reuptake inhibitor, is more expensive, but avoids the anticholinergic side-effects of the TCAs.

Zopiclone and zolpidem

These two hypnotics act on sub-units of the benzodiazepine receptors. They both have short half-lives, zopiclone 5 hours and zolpidem 2.5 hours. It has been suggested that they are likely to cause less dependence than the older benzodiazepine drugs, and do not cause rebound insomnia.

Barbiturates

Although barbiturates, and chloral hydrate in particular, continue to be prescribed, there is little reason for doing so in primary care. The drugs are toxic in overdose and cause dependence.

Herbal remedies

Almonds, camomile, catmint, fennel, ginseng, hops, indian hemp, lettuce, lime, marjoram, may blossom, melissa, mullein, oats, orange blossom, passion flower, poppy seed, rosemary, willow and valerian are all traditionally thought to be sedatives.

WHEN TO REFER

Few patients with insomnia alone in UK primary care will be referred for a specialist opinion, although in the US, specialist sleep clinics have been established. Unusual causes for insomnia which would indicate the need for referral include obstructive sleep apnoea and periodic limb movements in sleep. Both conditions are easier to diagnose with a history from the bed partner.

QUESTIONS FOR PARTNER WHO SHARES THE BEDROOM

- Does your partner stop breathing during the night? (Does this happen every night? How often does it happen?)
- Does your partner snore, gasp or make choking sounds during the night? (Does this happen every night? How often does it happen?)
- Do your partner's legs twitch, jerk, or kick during the night? (Does this happen every night? How often does it happen?)
- Have you noticed any recent changes in your partner's mood or emotional state?
- Has your partner's consumption of alcohol, nicotine, caffeine or other drugs changed recently?
- What do you think is the cause of your partner's difficulty in sleeping?

(Shapiro, 1993)

Obstructive sleep apnoea is associated with snoring and being overweight. It results in night-time awakenings and/or daytime sleepiness. Periodic limb movements in sleep describes rhythmical jerking movements of the legs – usually both legs are affected with joints flexing at 20–40 second intervals. Symptoms are worse in the first half of the night and may prevent sleep becoming established or cause the patient to wake up.

REFERENCES

Hauri P (1979). Behavioural treatment of insomnia. *Medical Times* **107**: 36–47.

Kupfer DJ, Reynolds CF (1997). Management of insomnia. *New England Journal of Medicine* **336**:341–6.

Morgan K, Clarke D (1997). Risk factors for late-life insomnia in a representative general practice sample. *British Journal of General Practice* **47**:116–69.

Morin CM, Culbert JP, Schwartz SM (1994). Nonpharmacological interventions for insomnia: A meta-analysis of treatment efficacy. *American Journal of Psychiatry* **151(8):**1172–80.

Murtagh DR, Greenwood KM (1995). Identifying effective psychological treatments for insomnia: a meta-analysis. *Journal of Consulting and Clinical Psychology* **63:**79–89.

Shapiro CM (1993). ABC of sleep disorders. BMJ Publishing Group, London.

Simon GE, VonKorff M (1997). Prevalence, burden and treatment of insomnia in primary care. *American Journal of Psychiatry* **154(10):**1417–23.

Stradling JR (1993). Recreational drugs and sleep. In *ABC of Sleep Disorders* (CM Shapiro ed). BMJ Publishing Group, London

FURTHER READING

Shapiro CM, Macfarlane JG, Hussain M (1994). *Conquering Insomnia*. Empowering Press, Toronto.

Sloan EP, Hauri P, Bootzin R (1993). The nuts and bolts of behavioural treatment for insomnia. *Journal of Psychosomatic Research* **37(suppl. 1):**19–37.

Nichol R (1996). *Sleep Like a Dream the Drug Free Way*. Sheldon Press, London.

SELF-HELP AND WEBSITES

National Sleep Foundation
www.sleepfoundation.org
A US site with information and advice about insomnia.

A Guide to Insomnia from 4anything.com
www.4insomnia.com
One of a series of practical guides.

NHS Direct – Sleeping Problems
www.healthcare.nhsdirect.nhs.uk
Provides insomnia advice and management.

chapter 8

The fatigued patient

IN THIS CHAPTER

- How to investigate the fatigued patient.
- Important diagnoses to consider in patients that are 'tired all the time'.
- Treatment options for chronic fatigue syndrome.

EPIDEMIOLOGY

Fatigue is common amongst patients in primary care (Table 8.1). There is a strong correlation between fatigue and psychological morbidity. The more severe the fatigue symptoms, the greater the chance of being a case on the General Health Questionnaire (GHQ). In a prospective study comparing patients presenting with viral illness, with matched controls, the strongest predictors of fatigue 6 months later were a past history of fatigue and psychological distress (Wessely *et al.*, 1995). In a search for predictors for post-viral fatigue, a cohort of primary care patients presenting with viral illness were followed for 6 months. Infective symptoms did not predict fatigue at 6 months, but psychiatric morbidity, belief in vulnerability to viruses and attributional style at interview were all associated with self-designated post-viral fatigue (Cope *et al.*, 1994).

Fatigue scores are normally distributed in the population and those with chronic severe symptoms probably represent the extreme range. Thus

---

Table 8.1. Epidemiology of fatigue

- In a community questionnaire survey (Pawlikowska *et al.*, 1994):
  – more than one-third self-reported substantial fatigue
  – in 18% the symptom duration was 6 months or longer
- Women are more likely to complain of fatigue than men, even after adjusting for psychological distress
- Only 1.4% of the patients with excessive tiredness attributed their symptoms to the chronic fatigue syndrome
- On an average GP's list, 360 patients might report excessive fatigue for more than 6 months, but only 3 would attribute their symptoms to the chronic fatigue syndrome

---

fatigue can be considered rather like hypertension where chronic fatigue does not represent a single diagnosis and the cut-off point is arbitrarily assigned. Unlike hypertension, however, the cut-off point does not imply benefit from treatment or have prognostic implications. The chronic fatigue syndrome is operationally defined (see below), but the label is only useful to define populations for research purposes. Patients who are severely disabled by their symptoms warrant further investigation and management, rather than restricting treatment to those satisfying arbitrary diagnostic criteria. It may, therefore, be more useful in primary care to describe the patient as suffering from 'chronic fatigue' rather than 'the chronic fatigue syndrome', which implies a greater degree of certainty than actually exists.

CHRONIC FATIGUE SYNDROME

Fatigue longer than 1 month is defined as prolonged fatigue; to diagnose chronic fatigue the symptoms must last 6 months or longer. The diagnosis is one of exclusion where physical examination and blood tests are normal and there is no history of melancholic depression (i.e. with loss of pleasure, morning awakening, guilt and anorexia), schizophrenia, eating disorder or alcohol abuse.

CRITERIA FOR CHRONIC FATIGUE SYNDROME

Unexplained fatigue which is not the result of ongoing exertion, not alleviated by rest and which results in a reduction in activity.

Plus four or more of the following symptoms:
- Impairment of memory or concentration.
- Sore throat.
- Tender cervical or axillary lymph nodes.
- Muscle pain.
- Polyarthralgia without swelling.
- Headaches of a new type, pattern or severity.
- Unrefreshing sleep.
- Post-exertional malaise lasting more than 24 hours.

Chronic fatigue has considerable morbidity. In a primary care cohort, only 28% of those identified as fatigued had recovered after 1 year. The mean score of the fatigued cohort on the Sickness Impact Profile of 11.3 is similar to that reported by patients with major medical illness (Kroenke et al., 1988).

IS IT POST-VIRAL FATIGUE?

There is little evidence to support the widely-held belief that chronic fatigue is usually post-viral. In one prospective cohort study, there was no evidence that common infective episodes in primary care were associated with chronic fatigue (Wessely et al., 1995). A second cohort study revealed a modest excess risk of fatigue 6 months after presenting with a viral illness of 1.45 (CI 1.14–2.04), but only in comparison to controls from another study (Cope et al., 1994). No consistent disorder of muscle function or persistent viral infection has been demonstrated.

MANAGEMENT IN PRIMARY CARE

'I'm tired all the time doctor.' Practitioners will be familiar with the sinking feeling associated with these words. Although almost any chronic disease or psychological illness can present as chronic fatigue, in the presence of a normal physical examination, laboratory testing is rarely helpful. In a prospective study of 405 patients with fatigue, less than 3% were found to have a partly medical diagnosis (Llewelyn, 1996). The following have been suggested as appropriate physical investigations for patient 'tired all the time':

SUGGESTED INVESTIGATIONS FOR CHRONIC FATIGUE

- Full blood count and erythrocyte sedimentation rate.
- B_{12} and folate.
- Biochemical profile.
- TFT.
- Glucose.
- Creatinine kinase (where myalgia is a dominant feature).
- Antinuclear antibody (where arthralgia is a dominant feature).

Although medical diagnoses are unusual, psychological diagnoses are common. In a community survey, Pawlikowska et al. (1994) reported that 60% of patients reporting fatigue of more than 6 months duration were cases on the GHQ, rising to 80% in those more severely affected.

In any patient presenting with medically unexplained fatigue (normal examination and blood screen), the main diagnoses to consider in addition to chronic fatigue syndrome are:

- ✓ Psychiatric disorders.
- ✓ Fibromyalgia.
- ✓ Post-glandular fever fatigue.

PSYCHIATRIC DISORDERS

The main psychiatric disorders to be considered are:

■ Depression.
■ Panic disorder.
■ Somatization.
■ Sleep disorder.

More than one psychiatric disorder may be present.

FIBROMYALGIA

There is a considerable overlap between chronic fatigue syndrome and fibromyalgia. Fibromyalgia is thought to affect 5% of the population and there is often a considerable delay in the diagnosis. It occurs predominantly in women and presents with a variable symptom complex of widespread musculoskeletal pain, severe fatigue, and multisystem 'functional disturbance'. The diagnosis is based on the typical symptom complex with negative investigations and characteristic multiple symmetrical hyperalgesic tender sites. Patients with chronic fatigue, tension headache, irritable bowel syndrome may also be suffering from fibromyalgia.

COMMON SYMPTOMS OF FIBROMYALGIA

■ Pain:
  – predominantly axial (neck and back),
  – may be morning stiffness and 'pain all over',
  – unresponsive to simple analgesia non-steroidal anti-inflammatory drugs .
■ Fatigue.

Continued on page 176

Common symptoms of fibromyalgia (*continued*)

■ Other:
  – subjective swollen extremities,
  – parasthesia or dysthesia of the hands and feet,
  – waking unrefreshed,
  – poor concentration/forgetfulness,
  – low mood, irritable,
  – headache,
  – diffuse abdominal pain,
  – urinary frequency/urgency.

(Doherty, 1993)

The prognosis of fibromyalgia, like other fatigue syndromes, is poor and management consists of sympathetic consultation and explanation of the condition. Low-dose TCAs and a graded exercise programme may also be helpful. A useful patient information sheet is produced by the Arthritis and Rheumatism Council.

POST-GLANDULAR FEVER FATIGUE

In contrast to generic 'post-viral fatigue' there is evidence from a prospective primary care cohort study of post-glandular fever fatigue. Excess fatigue was identified both in subjects with serologically proven glandular fever and those with a glandular fever-like illness with negative serology. The overall symptom complex was similar to that found in other fatigue syndromes, with the exception of hypersomnia, in contrast to insomnia. An empirical description of the syndrome was derived from interview data (White *et al.*, 1995):

FATIGUE SYNDROME ASSOCIATED WITH GLANDULAR FEVER-LIKE ILLNESSES

- Physical fatigue, particularly post-exertion.
- Mental fatigue.
- Hypersomnia.
- Retardation and poor concentration.
- Anhedonia.
- Irritability and emotional lability.

MANAGEMENT OF CHRONIC FATIGUE

The principles of treatment are similar to those used in the treatment of patients with somatic symptoms (see page 146).

THERAPEUTIC APPROACHES FOR CHRONIC FATIGUE SYNDROME

- Therapeutic consultations.
- Graded exercise programme.
- Antidepressants.
- Cognitive behaviour therapy (CBT).

The therapeutic consultation involves acknowledgement of the genuine nature of symptoms whilst not speculating on the aetiology. Try to ascertain the symptom type and its severity. An explanation of alternative causes of symptoms may be helpful, e.g. depression as a response to disability, or anxiety heightening awareness of somatic symptoms. Deal with unrealistic expectations of a 'cure' and emphasize that the goal of treatment is to improve function and minimize disability. Encourage the use of successful coping strategies whilst highlighting adverse strategies, e.g. excessive rest.

Antidepressants may be helpful, particularly when there are features of anxiety or depressive disorders. Sedative drugs, such as amitriptyline, can be used when insomnia is a feature, and should be commenced at low doses to prevent side-effects. Non-sedating compounds, such as lofepramine or imipramine, should be considered when fatigue is severe and sleep is less disturbed.

CBT is the most widely-used approach with good evidence of benefit in the secondary care setting. The model used is derived from that used in chronic pain and involves challenging attributions of illness. Typical cognitive distortions in chronic fatigue include:

- Depressive thought patterns.
- Anxiety provoking thought patterns.
- Fixed illness attributions.

A randomized controlled trial of 160 patients with chronic fatigue syndrome, from primary care in London, indicated that CBT and counselling were of equivalent benefit at 3 and 6 months (Risdale *et al.*, 2001). Unfortunately, this study did not have a control, usual care group.

A graded exercise programme substantially improved measures of fatigue and physical functioning in patients with chronic fatigue.

PRIMARY CARE MANAGEMENT ASSOCIATED WITH ADVERSE PROGNOSIS

- Doctor/patient communication breakdown.
- Uncertainty of the doctor making a diagnosis.
- Repeated investigations and referrals.
- Early sick certification.

WHEN TO REFER

It is not necessary to refer patients for confirmation of chronic fatigue since there is no diagnostic test available to confirm or refute the symptom. Medical referral is unlikely to result in a holistic approach, but rather in a battery of unnecessary tests. Specific indications for referral are:

- Old age (chronic fatigue is rare in the elderly).
- Relevant foreign travel.
- Weight loss (chronic fatigue is usually associated with weight gain).
- Neurological signs.
- Documented pyrexia.
- Abnormal investigations.

REFERENCES

Cope H, David A, Pelosi A, Mann A (1994). Predictors of chronic 'postviral' fatigue. *Lancet* **344(8926)**:864–8.

Doherty M (1993). *Practical Problems: Fibromyalgia Syndrome.* Arthritis and Rheumatism Council, Chesterfield.

Llewelyn MB (1996). Assessing the fatigued patient. *British Journal of Hospital Medicine* **55(3)**:125–9.

Kroenke K, Wood DR, Mangelsdorff AD, Meier NJ, Powell JB (1988). Chronic fatigue in primary care. Prevalence, patient characteristics and outcome. *Journal of the American Medical Association* **260(7)**:929–34.

Pawlikowska T, Chalder T, Hirsch SR, Wallace P, Wright DJ, Wessely SC (1994). Population based study of fatigue and psychological distress. *British Medical Journal* **308(6931)**:763–6.

Ridsdale L, Godfrey E, Chalder T, Seed P, King M, Wallace P, Wessely S, Fatigued Trialists Group (2001). Chronic fatigue in general practice: Is counselling as good as cognitive behavioural therapy. *British Journal of General Practice* **51**:19–24.

Wessely S, Chalder T, Hirsch S, Pawlikowska T, Wallace P, Wright DJ (1995). Postinfectious fatigue: prospective cohort study in primary care. *Lancet* **345(8961)**:1333–8.

White PD, Thomas JM, Amess J, Grover SA, Kangro HO, Clare AW (1995). The existence of a fatigue syndrome after glandular fever. *Psychological Medicine* **25**:907–16.

FURTHER READING

Doherty M (1993). *Practical Problems: Fibromyalgia Syndrome.* Chesterfield, Arthritis and Rheumatism Council.

WEBSITES

There are a large number of UK and US websites found by searching under 'chronic fatigue'. These often offer a particular perspective on the syndrome, its cause and possible treatment.

SELF-HELP

Arthritis and Rheumatism Council
ARC Cards Ltd, Brunel Drive, Northern Road Industrial Estate, Newark NG24 2DE
Produces patient information sheets on fibromyalgia.

chapter 9

The pregnant and post-partum patient

IN THIS CHAPTER

- Use of antidepressants in pregnancy and during lactation.
- Recognition and treatment of post–partum psychosis.
- Screening for postnatal depression.
- Treatment of postnatal depression.

INTRODUCTION

Mood and anxiety disorders are common during childbearing years. In this chapter the pregnant and the post-partum patient will be considered separately. It has been suggested that pregnancy is protective against psychiatric disorders; however, there is a clear risk of relapse in women who discontinue prophylactic psychotropic medication. There is an increased risk of psychiatric disorder in the first 3 months post-partum, although no increased incidence in the full year post-partum.

THE PREGNANT PATIENT

✓ Risk factors for depression.
✓ Antidepressant prescribing.

The commonest mental disorder in pregnancy is depression. The incidence of depression in pregnancy is probably about the same as in non-pregnant women; some women, however, are at increased risk.

RISK FACTORS FOR DEPRESSION IN PREGNANCY

- Prior history of depression.
- Younger age.
- Limited social support.
- Living alone.
- Greater number of children.
- Marital conflict.
- Ambivalence about pregnancy.

(Altshuler *et al.*, 1998)

For pregnant women on antidepressant medication, the risk of continuing with medication needs to be set against the risk of depressive relapse. It is important that depressive disorders in pregnancy are adequately treated because they are associated with:

- Inadequate prenatal care.
- Poor nutrition.
- Obstetric complications.
- Post-partum depression.

Management in primary care

In that it is best to avoid medication in pregnancy, consideration of psychological and social interventions should be the first approach. However, this should not be at the expense of ensuring that the depression is adequately treated. If medication is necessary, the following general points apply:

KEY POINTS: ANTIDEPRESSANT PRESCRIBING IN PREGNANCY

- Only prescribe if necessary.
- Avoid drug treatment in the first trimester if possible.
- Avoid new drugs.
- Use the lowest effective dose.
- Conception when on an antidepressant medication is not a reason for abortion.
- Lithium is the only antidepressant with a known increased risk to the foetus.

Neonatal withdrawal symptoms may occur, e.g. jitteriness, hyperexcitability; consider a tapered withdrawal over the last 4 weeks of pregnancy. If a pregnant women is currently well but has a history of relapse on withdrawal of medication, or if her current depression is moderate/severe, the benefits of medication usually outweigh the potential risks to the infant.

Table 9.1. Which drugs to prescribe in pregnancy

Fluoxetine: data from over 1000 pregnancies has shown no increased risk of malformations

Paroxetine and sertraline: in a prospective study of 267 women, there were no increased risks of foetal harm compared with controls

TCAs: there are no formal studies, but their use reviewed in 300 000 live births show no increase in foetal malformations

Avoid MAOIs

Avoid newer antidepressants

Avoid lithium

(Adapted from Bazire, 1999)

Bipolar and psychotic disorders

Where possible, patients with a bipolar disorder should be drug free for the first trimester. Lithium, carbamazepine and sodium valproate are associated with congenital abnormalities. Lithium is particularly associated with Ebstein's abnormality of the tricuspid valve (10–20 times the risk in the general population where it occurs in 1 in 20 000 cases). Spina bifida occurs in 0.5–1.0% of babies exposed to carbamazepine in the first trimester, and in 1–5% of those exposed to sodium valproate, compared to 0.03% in the general population. If accidental exposure has occurred, folate supplements may reduce the risk of neural tube defects and appropriate screening and scanning should be arranged (Austin and Mitchell, 1998).

Antipsychotic drugs may be associated with a small increased risk of congenital abnormalities following exposure in the first trimester. No evidence has shown such a risk with trifluoperazine. If antipsychotic drugs are indicated, switch to the minimum oral effective dose of trifluoperazine and ensure the patient receives intensive obstetric and psychiatric follow up.

When to refer

The usual principles about referring patients with depression apply. A lower threshold for referral might apply because of the desire to ensure a speedy recovery and the need to access psychological and social treatments. All patients with a bipolar or psychotic disorder should be referred if pregnant or planning pregnancy.

THE POST-PARTUM PATIENT

Epidemiology

Table 9.2 gives the epidemiology of post-partum psychosis. It is important to differentiate between normal post-partum reactions such as post-partum 'blues' and other more severe disorders that can be disabling and impair mothering ability. There are three main disorders to consider:

Table 9.2. Epidemiology of post-partum psychosis

- Incidence 1.5 per 1000 deliveries
- Risk factors:
  - family history
  - previous history of severe mental illness (risk 20–50%)
  - primagravida
- Little evidence for psychological causation

✓ Post-partum blues.
✓ Post-partum psychosis.
✓ Post-natal depression.

Post-partum blues

'Baby blues' are said to occur in about 50% of women, and are characterized by transitory emotional distress occurring between the third and tenth day post-partum and usually lasting for about 2 or 3 days.

POST-PARTUM BLUES: SYMPTOMS

Tearfullness.
Irritability.
Low mood.
Sleeplessness.
Poor concentration.
Distant feelings towards the infant.

Management in primary care

Post-partum 'blues' are normally monitored by the mother's family/partner and are reviewed by the midwife or health visitor. Mothers and families should be given appropriate reassurance. If the condition persists beyond a few days and is increasing in severity, a medical assessment should be made to consider a post-partum psychosis or postnatal depression.

Post-partum psychosis

The onset of post-partum psychosis is usually within the first 2 weeks following delivery, but rarely in the first 2 days.

CLINICAL FEATURES OF POST-PARTUM PSYCHOSIS

70% affective presentation.
25% schizophrenic presentation.
5% confusional state.

70% full recovery.
20% risk of future puerperal episodes.
50% risk of future psychotic episodes.

Poor prognosis is associated with a family history of serious mental illness, schizophrenia, neurotic personality and marital disharmony.

Management in primary care

Patients with post-partum psychosis need immediate referral to secondary care, using the Mental Health Act if necessary. The highest priority must be given to ensuring that the baby is safe.

Treatment in secondary care

An inpatient psychiatric admission may be necessary, ideally to a specialist mother and baby unit. However, this should not be regarded as routine. In recent years there has been a growth in the UK of community mental health services, which provide an alternative to admission. Such teams when linked in with intensive home support workers may be able to support the mother at home, particularly if she has a supportive social network of family and friends.

Mother and baby units

Ideally the mother and baby should be admitted to a specialist unit, and not the mother alone to an adult inpatient ward. Such an admission:

- Hopefully prevents prolonged separation that could adversely effect bonding between the mother and child.
- Allows the mother the opportunity for drug treatment and rest with supervised access to her child.
- Allows for the assessment of maternal competence.
- Allows for the assessment of potential harm or neglect to the child as the mother may have poor concentration or be responding to delusional thinking.
- Allows the mother to restore her sleep pattern whilst the child is looked after at night.

Child protection

Local authority social services departments may wish to hold a child protection case conference if there are any concerns regarding the safety and welfare of the baby. The Children Act places a very high priority on all those professionals involved with the child and the family to attend such conferences. Occasionally, it may be be necessary to make an application under the Children Act for an Emergency Placement Order (EPO). Such an application is normally made by a social worker, but can be made by any adult. When an EPO application is made to a magistrate, the child's parents are normally given 72 hours notice of the application and can appeal against such an order. In rare circumstances, a magistrate may grant an immediate order. The order can run for 7 days and be extended to a maximum of 14 days.

Post-natal depression

ICD-10 states that a depressive disorder to be truly post-partum should have an onset within 6 weeks post-delivery. Presentations after this period should be considered as mood disorders. In recent years, however, the post-partum period has become stretched to the extent that many people now refer to depression within the first year of childbirth as a post-partum disorder. Epidemiology of post-natal depression is shown in Table 9.3.

Table 9.3. Epidemiology of post-natal depression

- Incidence 10% in the first year
- Greatest incidence in the first 3 months
- Episodes typically last 2–6 months

Risk factors
- Previous depression
- Obstetric complications in vulnerable women
- Psychosocial adversity:
  – stressful life events
  – unemployment
  – lack of supportive relationships
  – youth
- Premature or unwell baby

Diagnosis and recognition

The clinical features of post-natal depression are not distinctive, but reflect a diagnosis of depression:

- Low mood.
- Depressive thoughts.

- Excessive crying (the amount and intensity may be a pointer to the potential seriousness of the episode).
- Anhedonia – no enjoyment from the infant.
- Sleeplessness (outside night-time care duties).
- Anxiety and excessive worry over the child's health.
- Exhaustion, lack of energy, psychomotor retardation and hypersomnia.
- Inability to meet childcare and household duties.
- Reduced/poor concentration.
- Decreased libido.
- Worsening relationships, increasing irritability leading to hostility and possible aggression.
- Suicidal and infanticidal thoughts are rare but need to be assessed:
  'Any thoughts of harming yourself?'
  'Any thoughts of harming the baby?'

Screening

Some areas have introduced health visitor screening for post-natal depression using the Edinburgh Post-natal Depression Scale (EPDS; Figure 9.1, overleaf) (Cox *et al.*, 1987). Health visitors will be familiar with this scale which is a simple ten-point questionnaire (scored 0–3), which the health visitor may complete with the mother. A cut off of 12/13 indicates probability of depression. In a community sample, the EPDS had a specificity of 92.5% and a sensitivity of 88%. Thus the likelihood ratio is 12.

Pre-test probability 10% (screening)	Positive (12+) implies a post-test probability of depression of 60%
Pre-test probability 50% (surgery)	Positive (12+) implies a post-test probability of depression of 93%

The scale can also be reused to assess how the mother's mental state is responding to treatment.

EDINBURGH POST-NATAL DEPRESSION SCALE

As you have recently had a baby, we would like to know how you are feeling. Please tick (✓) the appropriate boxes which come closest to how you have felt IN THE PAST 10 DAYS, not just how you feel today. Here is an example, I have felt happy:

Yes, all the time ☐
Yes, most of the time ☑
No, not very often ☐
No, not at all ☐

This would mean I have felt happy most of the time during the past week. Please complete the other questions in the same way.

In the past 7 days:

1. I have been able to laugh and see the funny side of things:
As much as I always could ☐
Not quite so much now ☐
Definitely not so much now ☐
Not at all ☐

2. I have looked forward with enjoyment to things:
As much as I ever did ☐
Rather less than I used to ☐
Definitely less than I used to ☐
Not at all ☐

3. I have blamed myself unnecessarily when things went wrong:
Yes, most of the time ☐
Yes, some of the time ☐
Not very often ☐
No, never ☐

4. I have been anxious or worried for no good reason:
No, not at all ☐
Hardly ever ☐
Yes, sometimes ☐
Yes, very often ☐

5. I have felt scared or panicky for no very good reason:
Yes, quite a bit ☐
Yes, sometimes ☐
No, not much ☐
No, not at all ☐

6. Things have been getting on top of me:
Yes, most of the time I haven't been able to cope at all ☐
Yes, sometimes I haven't been coping as well as usual ☐
No, most of the time I have coped quite as well ☐
No, I have been coping as well as ever ☐

7. I have been so unhappy that I have had difficulty sleeping:
Yes, most of the time ☐
Yes, sometimes ☐
Not very often ☐
No, not at all ☐

8. I have felt sad or miserable:
Yes, most of the time ☐
Yes, quite often ☐
Not very often ☐
No, not at all ☐

9. I have been so unhappy that I have been crying:
Yes, most of the time ☐
Yes, quite often ☐
Only occasionally ☐
No, never ☐

10. The thought of harming myself has occurred to me:
Yes, quite often ☐
Sometimes ☐
Hardly ever ☐
Never ☐

Figure 9.1. Edinburgh Post-natal Depression Scale.

Management in primary care
Support from GP and health visitor

Controlled studies of psychological treatments delivered by nurses have shown improvement in maternal mood compared with routine care. In mothers with post-natal depression, non-directive counselling by health visitors (nine sessions over 3 months) was more effective at improving mood than an untreated control group (Holden *et al.*, 1989). Again in mothers with post-natal depression, six sessions of CBT-based counselling by health visitors was more effective than one session, and equally effective as fluoxetine (Appleby *et al.*, 1997).

Drug treatment

Antidepressants have the same role and benefit in post-natal depression as in non-post-natal depression (Table 9.4). There is no evidence to support the use of progesterone. Oestrogen has been shown in one study to be of benefit in severe chronic cases.

Prophylactic antidepressants given immediately after a subsequent birth have been shown to greatly reduce relapse rates.

Table 9.4. Use of antidepressants during lactation

- For all antidepressants, the amount excreted in breast milk is low and unlikely to cause neonatal toxicity

- TCAs (first choice): amitriptyline and imipramine, very low levels (0.1% maternal dose) appearing in milk – unlikely to be of harm

- SSRIs (if risk of overdose): sertraline or paroxetine is probably the drug of choice
  - sertraline: not known to be harmful (BNF comment)
  - paroxetine: no detectable drug in breast-fed infants
  - fluoxetine: avoid, significant amounts in breast milk (BNF comment)
  - citalopram: use with caution (BNF comment)

- Avoid MAOIs and newer antidepressants

- Observe infants for drowsiness, jitteriness, especially if small

CASE STUDY: COLLETTE

Collette is a 34-year-old mother of two, married to Paul who works during the week at the Paris office of an advertising agency. Until the birth of her first child 2 years ago, Collette was a senior partner in a London-based corporate advertising agency. Collette gave birth to Rachel in October 1997 and planned to return to work in the spring of the following year, having spent several months of 'quality parenting' with her daughter. In April of 1998, Collette found that she was pregnant again and negotiated a career break from work. In November, she gave birth to Guy.

Although disappointed about not returning to work, Collette was overjoyed with her two young children and devoted her entire energy to them. Paul spoke to Collette every evening and came home at weekends, sometimes taking long weekend breaks. By the time that Guy was 5 months old and Rachel was starting to toddle and be into everything, Collette began to lose her sense of purpose and drive. She began to get less pleasure from the children, was often tired and lacking in energy. She began to go out less and neglect her appearance, some days not even bothering to dress. The area in which they lived was something of a commuter dormitory and Collette had few community supports.

On returning home from Paris one Friday evening, Paul found the house cold and unlit. The sink was full of washing up and the remnants of several take-away meals were evident. The children were in grubby night attire. Collette had obviously been crying.

Paul called out the GP who prescribed an antidepressant and recommended that Paul took some time off to look after Collette and the children. The health visitor called a couple of times over the next fortnight, and Collette's mother came to help once Paul had returned to work. Collette was put in touch with a self-help post-natal support group. Collette's mood improved slowly over a 3-month period.

Lessons from the case study

- Depression in the months following childbirth often requires standard treatment.
- Use of medication and social interventions.
- Health visitors are a very important resource.
- Depression is no respector of social class.
- Need to ensure children are looked after.

When to refer

The great majority of mothers with post-natal depression are treated by the primary health care team without specialist referral. However, there are occasions when it is appropriate to refer to secondary care and where shared care might be beneficial.

WHEN TO REFER

- When depression is severe and/or not responding to simple measures.
- When there is risk of self-harm or harm to the child.
- When there is a need to access specialist psychological or social interventions.

REFERENCES

Altshuler LL, Hendrick V, Cohen LS (1998). Course of mood and anxiety disorders during pregnancy and the post partum period. *Journal of Clinical Psychiatry* **59(2)**:29–32.

Appleby L, Warner R, Whitton A, Faragher B (1997). A controlled study of fluoxetine, and cognitive behavioural counselling in the treatment of postnatal depression. *British Medical Journal* **314**:932–6.

Austin MV, Mitchell PB (1998). Psychotropic medications in pregnant women. *Medical Journal of Australia* **169**:428–31.

Bazire S (1999). *Psychotropic Drug Directory.* Mark Allen Publishing, Salisbury.

Cox JL, Holden JM, Sogovsky R (1987). Detection of postnatal depression. Development of the 10 item Edinburgh Postnatal Depression Scale. *British Journal of Psychiatry* **150**:782–6.

Holden JM, Sagovsky R, Cox JL (1989). Counselling in a general practice setting: a controlled study of health visitor intervention in the treatment of postnatal depression. *British Medical Journal* **298**:223–6.

FURTHER READING

Cooper PJ, Murray L (1998). Postnatal depression. *British Medical Journal* **316**:1884–6.

Marshall F (1994). *Coping with Postnatal Depression.* Sheldon Press, London.

Sapsted AM (1994). *Banish Baby Blues.* Harper Collins, Glasgow.

WEBSITES

www.mentalhealth.com

This is a huge English-language website based in Canada, which contains masses of information across the range of mental health problems and provides many useful links to other sites. Some of the linked chat sites are American.

SELF-HELP

Association for Postnatal Illness

25 Jerdan Place, Fulham, London SW6 1BE

Tel: 020 7386 0868

Fax: 020 7386 8885

A national network of telephone and postal volunteers who themselves have had and recovered from post-natal depression. The association aims to support and educate women suffering from post-natal depression, increase public awareness of the illness and encourages research into its cause and nature. The association also provides counselling and telephone advice as well as leaflets, booklets, a newsletter and specialist publications for health care professionals.

Cry-sis
London WC1N 3XX
Tel: 020 7404 5011
For help and support with a crying baby.

Home Start UK
2 Salisbury Road, Leicester LE1 7QR
Tel: 0116 233 9955
Fax: 0116 233 0232
Home Start UK volunteers offer regular support, friendship and practical help to young families with at least one child under five, who are experiencing difficulties and stress. Volunteers visit families in their own homes helping to prevent family crisis and breakdown.

Meet-a-mum
c/o Mrs Briony Hallam, 14 Willis Road, Croydon, Surrey CR0 2XX
Helpline: 020 8768 0123
Self-help groups for mothers with small children.

National Childbirth Trust
Alexandra House, Oldham Terrace, London W3 6NH
Tel: 020 8992 8637
Runs antenatal classes (fee charged) and provides breastfeeding counsellors and organizes a network of local post-natal groups.

chapter 10

The patient with an eating disorder

IN THIS CHAPTER

- Detection of eating disorders – difference from normal dieting.
- Assessment in primary care.
- Early management of eating disorders in primary care.

EPIDEMIOLOGY

The epidemiology of eating disorders is shown in Table 10.1.

Table 10.1. Epidemiology of eating disorders

- Prevalence in young women:
  - anorexia nervosa 0.5%
  - bulimia nervosa 1–2%
  - partial syndrome eating disorders 5%
- Risk factors:
  - mean age of onset 15/16 years
  - women (x10)
  - family history of weight disorder or mood disorder
  - alcohol/substance misuse
  - social groups, e.g. dancers, athletes
  - insulin-dependent diabetes
  - history of sexual abuse
  - dieting
  - ?enmeshed over-protective family relationships
- Suicide rate anorexia nervosa x32
- Overall mortality anorexia nervosa x5

In adolescent girls, eating disorders are the third most common disorder behind obesity and asthma. Rates for males are about 5–10% those for females. The prevalence of eating disorders is directly related to rates of dieting behaviour, although only a minority of young people who diet go on to develop an eating disorder. When dieting and the desire to be thin combine with problems of self-esteem and interpersonal relationships, an eating disorder is a possible outcome.

NATURAL HISTORY OF ANOREXIA AND BULIMIA

Anorexia nervosa
A review of long-term outcome (20 years) suggests 50% of patients make a good recovery with normalization of three outcome parameters: weight, menstrual pattern and eating behaviour, 30% have a fair outcome (improvement in one or two parameters), and 20% have a poor outcome (no improvement or death). However, most patients remain impaired in physical and social functioning, and continue to have disordered eating practices.

Bulimia nervosa
The outcome of bulimia nervosa is less well described. In intermediate term studies, about 20% of patients continued to have bulimia after 2–5 years, a further 25% still had bulimic symptoms.

Prognostic factors
For both anorexia nervosa and bulimia nervosa, poorer prognosis is associated with lower initial minimum weight, failure to respond to previous treatments, premorbidly disturbed family relationships and severe personality disorder. For anorexia nervosa, the presence of vomiting is a poor prognostic feature and, for bulimia nervosa, the use of purgatives.

(Wilhelm and Clarke, 1998)

RECOGNITION AND DIAGNOSIS

The two main eating disorder diagnoses are anorexia nervosa and bulimia nervosa. The diagnostic features are set out below.

DIAGNOSIS: ANOREXIA NERVOSA

- Weight loss (body mass index (BMI)★ 17.5 or less).
- Self-induced weight loss by avoidance of fattening foods; may also vomit, purge or exercise.
- Body image distortion – the patient believes herself to be overweight.
- Amenorrhoea or delayed puberty.

$$\star BMI = \frac{weight\ (kg)}{height^2\ (m^2)}$$

DIAGNOSIS: BULIMIA NERVOSA

- Binge eating, characterized by eating a large amount within a short period of time, associated with loss of control.
- Behaviours to counteract the weight gain, e.g. self-induced vomiting and laxative misuse.
- Morbid fear of fatness.

Partial syndrome eating disorders are more common than the full-blown syndromes. In partial syndrome disorders, patients either have weight loss or binge eating, but not necessarily the full clinical picture.

Approximately half of cases of bulimia and partial syndrome eating disorders remain 'hidden' in primary care (Whitehouse *et al.*, 1992). As with depression, undetected disorders may reflect the less severe disorders. Indicators that might alert the GP to the presence of an eating disorder are set out below.

INDICATORS FOR THE GP

- Non-specific psychological complaints.
- Psychosomatic complaints.
- Concern to diet at normal weight.
- Past weight fluctuation.
- Past menstrual irregularity.
- Past psychiatric referral.
- Family psychiatric problems.
- Vegetarian diet.
- Failure to gain weight in pregnancy.

(King, 1990)

Relatives or friends may be the first contact – expressing concern about eating behaviours and/or weight loss. In that many girls go on a diet, how can a parent or GP distinguish between 'normal adolescent dieting' and early anorexia nervosa? Pointers to help distinguish between the two are set out below.

EARLY RECOGNITION OF ANOREXIA NERVOSA

Denial of dieting
- Most people on a diet will admit so readily and often want to talk about dieting: about different diets that others have tried, the amount of weight loss that would be expected and how much they have cheated.
- The girl with anorexia nervosa will often deny being on a diet.

Denial of hunger and craving
- People who are dieting will admit to feeling ravenous and admit to cravings for specific foods.
- Many anorexics will say they are not hungry and will be very reluctant to admit to desiring particular types of high-calorie food.

Covering-up weight loss

- 'Normal dieters' are delighted with their weight loss and talk about the number of pounds they have lost.
- The anorexic will often wear clothes to hide their weight loss, and in the early stages may say that they are not losing weight at all and that there is no cause for concern.

Increased interest in food

- Whilst an increased interest in food is common in most people who diet, the 'normal dieter' will try and avoid the temptation of food.
- In contrast, the anorexic often takes great pleasure in preparing, handling and cooking food for others.

Needing to eat less than others

- The 'normal dieter' does not appear to be particularly competitive with others in the family.
- In contrast, the anorexic always wants to have less food on her plate than other family members, particularly her sisters or mother. If she has prepared the food she will often give unrealistically large helpings to other family members.

Eating slowly

- 'Normal dieters' often eat rapidly, trying to satisfy their hunger and clearing everything from their plate.
- Anorexic girls will dawdle over eating, chew food for longer periods, push peas around on their plate and finish the meal long after others.

Increasing obsessionality and perfectionism

- Whilst these features may occur in anyone who is starving, they appear to occur early in those developing anorexia nervosa, as revealed in preciseness about meal times and the calorie content of food. Rules about eating are mirrored by increasing obsessionality in other areas of life, such as schoolwork and relationships.

Other behavioural changes
- The hoarding of food, night-time eating, becoming increasingly phobic about eating in public, increased exercise and the use of diuretics or laxatives.

(Freeman, 1999)

The following questions will help elicit whether or not a patient has an eating disorder:

- What is your current weight (weigh if necessary) and what is your ideal weight? Patients with an eating disorder will usually admit to an unrealistically low ideal weight. If the thin patient acknowledges she is underweight and would like to put on weight, the patient does not have anorexia nervosa.
- What do you eat on a typical day? What have you eaten over the past 24 hours? Is there evidence for severe restriction or chaotic eating?
- Ask the ways in which the patient tries to lose weight, e.g. self-induced vomiting, laxative use and exercise.
- Ask about loss of control of eating: 'When you are down do you ever eat more than you should?' and 'Some people under-eat when stressed, many over-eat. How does stress affect you?'
- What has happened to your periods?

MANAGEMENT IN PRIMARY CARE

The principles underpinning the management of eating disorders in primary care are, firstly, to establish a therapeutic relationship, secondly, to monitor and stabilize the current situation and, finally, to set jointly agreed goals for treatment. Freeman (1999) has set out more detailed advice about the management for anorexia nervosa and bulimia nervosa.

Anorexia nervosa

✓ Form a therapeutic alliance.
✓ Do not rush into specialist referral.
✓ Monitor food intake with a diary and get the patient's
   agreement to stabilize her weight.
✓ Identify serious physical concerns.
✓ Assess co-morbid psychiatric disorder.
✓ Provision of education and dietary advice.
✓ Advice to her family.

- Form a therapeutic alliance – include the family for younger patients.
- Do not rush into a specialist referral. Patients with anorexia are often very frightened of treatment. See the patient regularly to try and stabilize the situation and build up the patient's trust in treatment.
- Monitor food intake with a diary and get the patient's agreement to stabilize their weight.
- Identify serious physical concerns. Severe weight loss may cause several physical problems. Patients should therefore have:
  - a physical examination (bradycardia, hypotension, bruising),
  - biochemical screen including electrolytes, liver function tests and serum glucose,
  - full blood count (anaemia 15%, leucopenia 50%, thrombocytopenia 30%),
  - ECG (arrhythmias and ECG changes),
  - consider bone densitometry.
- Assess co-morbid psychiatric disorder: depressive disorders may be present and merit treatment.
- Provision of education and dietary advice:
  - give some simple educational information about dietary balance, what happens when periods stop and the long-term effects on bones in terms of osteoporosis,
  - it is well worth pointing out that if the girl has not finished growing, that as well as ending up slimmer, she will also end up shorter for growth is definitely stunted by anorexia nervosa,

- give some simple dietary advice, such as not counting calories and trying to eat small regular meals spaced out during the day, rather than starving during the day and only eating in the evening.
- Advice to the family:
  - with the patient's permission, give some advice to the family,
  - topics that may be briefly covered include: families are not 'to blame' for anorexia nervosa and it is a psychological condition with no single cause.

Bulimia nervosa

✓ Acknowledge the disorder.
✓ Keeping a diary.
✓ Assess mood and suicide risk.
✓ Beginning to make changes.
✓ Techniques to avoid bingeing.
✓ Self-help.
✓ Drug treatment.

- Acknowledge the disorder:
  - reassurance that the disorder is common, that many women suffer from it and that treatment is available may all help,
  - the patient with bulimia may have fears of rejection; of being told to pull herself together or that the GP will be repulsed by her behaviour.
- Keeping a diary:
  - introduce the idea of a diary and stress that for the first week or two you do not want the behaviour to change,
  - the purpose of the diary is to record eating as accurately as possible – the number of times she binges and vomits, what factors preceded the binge, where the binge occurred, what her feelings were, and how she felt afterwards,
  - the pattern of eating is often shown to be one of restricted intake preceding a binge followed by self-induced vomiting.

- Assess mood and suicide risk: depressive symptoms are common in bulimia nervosa. Usually, they are secondary to the bulimia though sometimes it is difficult to assess which came first.
- Beginning to make changes:
  - introduce the idea of dieting less strictly,
  - beginning to eat something, however small, in the morning rather than starving,
  - advise her to eat regular, albeit small, meals during the day – a breakfast, lunch, mid-afternoon snack and dinner to offset starvation during the day,
  - reassure her that this diet will not result in increased weight but rather spread the calories out more appropriately during the day.
- Techniques to avoid bingeing. Simple advice can be given about:
  - trying to eating in company,
  - decreasing the amount of food kept in the house,
  - not shopping when hungry,
  - using distractions such as exercise or phoning someone,
  - encouraging the patient to identify other 'distracting' activities she can use.
- Self-help: advice about manuals, self-help groups – self-help alone is effective in about 20% of women.
- Drug treatment: fluoxetine 60 mg/day has been shown to reduce the frequency of binge eating and self-induced vomiting.

A comparison between medication, CBT and combined treatment is given in Table 10.2 (overleaf).

Table 10.2. Effect sizes for medication, CBT and combined treatment

Outcome	No. of studies	Overall weighted effect size (95% CI)
Medication trials:		
Binge frequency	9	0.66 (0.52–0.81)
Purge frequency	6	0.39 (0.24–0.54)
Depression	9	0.73 (0.58–0.88)
CBT trials:		
Binge frequency	17	1.28 (1.09–1.47)
Purge frequency	24	1.22 (1.06–1.39)
Depression	19	1.31 (1.10–1.51)
Combined treatment:		
Binge frequency	4	1.77 (1.34–2.21)
Purge frequency	5	1.33 (0.94–1.73)

(Whittal *et al.*, 1999)

CASE STUDY: JENNIFER

Dr Jones is not surprised that Jennifer is booked into his morning surgery. Jennifer is 24 and has a 2-year-old son (Matthew). She suffered from post-natal depression following the birth of Matthew and she remains on fluoxetine 20 mg. She attends the surgery regularly complaining of tiredness, occasional dizziness and low mood. Jennifer is of normal weight but has discussed diets with Dr Jones in the past. He knows that she attends a local weight-watchers group.

Jennifer is accompanied to the consultation by her husband who informs Dr Jones that he has discovered that Jennifer has been bingeing food and then causing herself to vomit. Jennifer also admits to using over-the-counter laxatives.

Dr Jones arranges to see Jennifer again on her own and finds out that the eating disorder has been present for about the last 18 months. She became more concerned about her weight following her pregnancy. She describes a difficult marital relationship since the birth of the baby. She feels ashamed of her eating pattern and wants to stop it. Dr Jones asks Jennifer to keep a food diary which she does over the next 2 weeks (Figure 10.1, overleaf).

Dr Jones reviews the food diary with Jennifer and points out how the binges follow episodes of severe restriction. Information is given about spreading calories throughout the day, reassurance given that this will not lead to marked weight gain. Information also given that weight fluctuates around a mean and that 2 or 3 pounds either side of such an average is normal. Jennifer returns 2 weeks later feeling reasonably pleased only having had one binge. She still describes feeling low, however, and continues to complain that her husband is unsupportive. Dr Jones decides to increase the fluoxetine to 60 mg and recommends that Jennifer and her husband attend Relate for marital counselling.

Lessons from the case study

- Dieting when normal weight.
- Eating disorder presents with psychological symptoms.
- Bulimia often occurs with depression.
- Management of bulimia with a simple food diary and advice.
- Use of medication.
- Use of psychosocial interventions.
- No immediate referral necessary.

	Breakfast	Mid-morning snack	Lunch	Mid-afternoon snack	Dinner	Evening
Monday	Black coffee	–	Pkt crisps, apple	3 pkts biscuits, cake (vomit)	–	–
Tuesday	Toast, black coffee	–	Sandwich, apple	–	Chicken and salad	–
Wednesday	Black coffee	–	Tuna pasta	–	Tuna pasta	Binge and vomit
Thursday	Could not complete diary – binge x2 – vomit and use of laxatives					
Friday	Black coffee, crispbread	–	Sandwich, apple	–	Chicken and salad	–
Saturday	Apple, black coffee	–	Sandwich, fruit salad	Half-litre ice-cream, 3 bowls of cornflakes, 1 cake (vomit)	–	–
Sunday	Pear, black coffee	–	Salad and trout	–	Roast lamb, vegetables (no potatoes)	–

Figure 10.1. Jennifer's food diary.

WHEN TO REFER

- Anorexia nervosa:
  - rapid weight loss,
  - BMI 16 or less,
  - physical complications,
  - marked vomiting or laxative abuse,
  - simple interventions have failed.
- Bulimia nervosa:
  - simple interventions have failed,
  - marked depressed mood,
  - concurrent substance misuse, self-harming,
  - need to access specialist psychological treatments.

WHAT TO EXPECT FROM SECONDARY CARE

- Diagnosis and risk assessment.
- Specific treatment programmes for anorexia may include specialist inpatient and/or day patient facilities.
- Access to specialist psychological treatments, including family therapy for younger patients.
- Admission under the Mental Health Act may be necessary for severe anorexia nervosa.

REFERENCES

Freeman C (1999). *Eating Disorders: A Guide for Primary Care*. Psychiatry 2000, Wyeth Pharmaceuticals, Guildford.

King MB (1990). Eating disorders in general practice. *Journal of Royal Society of Medicine* **83**:229–32.

Whitehouse AM, Cooper PJ, Vize CV, Hill C, Vogel L (1992). Prevalence of eating disorders in three Cambridge general practices. *British Journal of General Practice* **42**:57–60.

Wilhelm KA, Clarke SD (1998). Eating disorders from a primary care perspective. *Medical Journal of Australia Practice Essentials* **168**:458–63.

Whittal ML, Agras WS, Gould RA (1999). Bulimia nervosa: a meta-analysis of psychosocial and pharmacological treatments. *Behaviour Therapy* **30**:117–35.

FURTHER READING

Schmitt U, Treasure J (1993). *Getting Better Bit(e) by Bit(e). A Survival Guide.* Lawrence Earlbaum Associates, London.
Fairburn C (1996). *Overcoming Binge Eating.* Guildford Press, New York.

WEBSITES

Academy for Eating Disorders
www.acadeatdis.org
Newsletters and information.

National Centre for Eating Disorders
www.eating-disorder.org.uk
Provides advice and information.

National Eating Disorder Information Centre (Canada)
www.nedic.on.ca
Provides advice and information.

SELF-HELP

Eating Disorders Association
Sackville Place, 44 Magdalen Street, Norwich, Norfolk NR3 1JU
Tel: 01603 621414 (helpline)
    01603 765050 (youth helpline 4 pm–6.30 pm)
    01603 619090 (administration)
Provides information packs for patients and professionals.

Eating Disorders Club
Stricklandgate House, 92 Stricklandgate, Kendal, Cumbria LA9 4PU
Tel: 01539 736077

chapter 11

The substance abuser

IN THIS CHAPTER

- Management of requests for drugs from temporary residents.
- Minimum standards of care for opiate users.
- Medical complications of opiate and stimulant misuse.
- Management of benzodiazepine withdrawal.
- Prescribing for controlled drugs.

INTRODUCTION

Shared care in the management of drug misusers is government policy in the UK, although strategies to implement shared care protocols are patchy (Geralda and Tighe, 1999). Department of Health (1999) guidelines distinguish between the generalist (a GP), the specialized generalist (a GP with a special interest in substance misuse) and the specialist, with roles and expectations varying according to expertise.

Many GPs would prefer to leave treatment of substance misuse to specialists, but many aspects of recognition, harm prevention and treatment of medical complications will remain in primary care.

Table 11.1. Epidemiology of substance misuse

- Age 16–29 years (peak age 20s):
  - 50% taken illegal substance at some time
  - 18% use in previous month
  - 5% two substances or more in previous month
- Male : female ratio 3:1
- Opiate misuse:
  - mortality x12
  - suicide rate x10
  - injecting users at particular risk

EPIDEMIOLOGY

Substance misuse is a significant and increasing problem for primary care (Table 11.1). It is no longer a problem confined to areas of urban deprivation. The total number of drug misusers presenting for treatment in the 6 months ending March 1998 was about 30 000 in Great Britain.

Although substance misuse conjures up images of illegal drugs, such as opiates and stimulants, prescribed drugs, particularly benzodiazepines, may cause dependence, whether obtained on prescription or from the street. In a substantial proportion of patients, drug misuse tends to improve with time and age.

MANAGEMENT IN PRIMARY CARE

✓ Temporary residents.
✓ Opiate misuse.
✓ Stimulant misuse.
✓ Benzodiazepine misuse.
✓ Prescribing controlled drugs.

Temporary residents

There is often a difference between known patients and temporary residents when considering the management of substance misuse. There needs to be a policy in place to avoid confrontations.

If unknown patients request drugs of abuse (see below) their identity needs to be established. If possible a check should be made to establish whether they have recently made similar requests to neighbouring practices. Although the counsel of perfection is not to prescribe, a consideration of personal and staff safety may mean prescriptions are given. If a decision is made to prescribe, only a small quantity should be prescribed, pending checking details.

DRUGS OF ABUSE

- Opiates (including codeine).
- Stimulants.
- Benzodiazepines.
- Anticholinergics.
- Chlormethiazole.
- Barbiturates.

CASE STUDY: TEMPORARY RESIDENT

The reception manager interrupted the Friday morning partners' meeting to ask for our help. A young man in his 20s was seeking to register as a temporary patient. He was just out of prison and wanted continuing supplies of drugs. He had already approached three other practices in the town all of whom had refused to take him on. He was smartly dressed, polite and tearful because of his difficulties. He was able to produce proof of identity, but not his medical card. The duty doctor agreed to see him at an early afternoon appointment allowing time for some routine checks. The practice manager quickly established, following three telephone calls to neighbouring practices, that he had been seen at another practice and prescribed medication earlier in the week. He was, in fact, registered at a different practice some 2 miles distant. We explained the situation to the staff at his own practice and arranged an appointment that evening. When he appeared for his appointment the duty doctor explained at the reception desk that we were unable to see him and that an appointment had been made at his own surgery. His pleasant demeanour rapidly evaporated, and he became abusive, swearing at the doctor and staff. He did, however, leave the building without recourse to the police. The health authority were informed and local practices circulated to avoid further problems.

Lessons from the case study

- Always ask the patient to confirm their identity – a medical card is ideal as it allows details to be checked with the registered practitioner and avoids the use of multiple aliases.
- If possible, check with local practices when there is suspicion of obtaining drugs for abuse.
- Those seeking drugs will often appear plausible. Do not be taken in by a seeming genuine story.
- Avoid confrontation if possible. This patient was advised in reception where a physical barrier existed between him and the staff. Always remain calm and composed. In this case, an appointment was made with his own GP and thus a 'helpful approach' was presented to the patient.
- Utilize local mechanisms to alert neighbouring practices.

For known patients, a therapeutic alliance may be established using the principles set out below.

OPIATE MISUSE

For GPs without a specialist interest in drug misuse, it is important to maintain a non-judgemental approach to patients who disclose any misuse. Patients with a history of opiate misuse may present for a variety of reasons unrelated to their drug use. A minimum assessment and a gold standard assessment are set out below.

MINIMUM ASSESSMENT OPIATE MISUSE

- Identification of medical and mental health problems that would merit specialist referral.
- Advice on harm minimization, in particular, immunization against hepatitis B and the risk of injecting.
- Assessing the motivation of the patient for seeking specialist help to reduce dependence.
- Notify the patient to the Regional Drug Misuse Database.

FULL ASSESSMENT OF OPIATE MISUSE

- Treat any emergency or acute problem.
- Confirm the patient is taking drugs (history, examination and urine analysis).
- Assess the degree of dependence.
- Identify the complications of drug misuse and assess risk behaviour.
- Identify other medical, social and mental health problems.
- Give advice on harm minimization including, if appropriate, access to sterile needles and syringes, testing for hepatitis and HIV, and immunization against hepatitis B.
- Determine the patient's expectations of treatment and the degree of motivation to change.
- Assess the most appropriate level of expertise required to manage the patient (this may alter over time) and refer/liaise appropriately.
- Determine the need for substitute medication — in the case of the generalist, this should be with advice, ideally through shared care structures.
- Notify the patient to the Regional Drug Misuse Database.

(Department of Health, 1999)

A risk assessment should include not only risk to self (psychotic symptoms and intrusive thoughts of self-harm merit psychiatric referral), but also risk to others. Any concerns about risk to children should be brought to the immediate attention of the local social services child care department.

The GP may be in a position to promote harm minimization which does not depend on specialist knowledge.

Harm reduction

- If using, reduce or stop injecting.
- If injecting, reduce or stop the sharing of equipment.
- If sharing, clean the equipment first.

Consider:
- Education about safer sex.
- Hepatitis B immunization.
- HIV testing.
- Local services needle exchange.

Management

No doctor should be pressurized into prescribing substitute medication. Indeed, the Department of Health (1999) recommendations are clear: *'only in exceptional circumstances should the decision to offer substitute medication without specialist generalist or specialist advice be made'*. Local protocols may be in place that set out opiate prescribing guidelines.

The medical complications of opiate misuse are set out in Table 11.2. All GPs need to be aware of these complications both to enable them to give appropriate health promotion advice and to recognize and treat complications as might arise.

Table 11.2. Medical complications of opiate misuse

Drug related
Side effects (e.g. constipation, hallucinations)
Overdose (e.g. respiratory depression)
Withdrawal (e.g. irritability, fits)

Route specific
Smoking (asthma)
Injecting (abscesses, cellulitis)

Sharing: needles, syringes and injection equipment
Hepatitis B and C, HIV and other blood-borne viruses

General
Anaemia, poor nutrition, poor dentition, deep vein thrombosis,
pulmonary emboli

Infections
Bacterial endocarditis, tuberculosis, septicaemia, pneumonia

Psychiatric problems
Psychotic features, suicidal behaviour, confusional states

Opiate withdrawal

The emergency treatment for opiate withdrawal will depend on locally agreed provision. There are a variety of drugs that can be used. Specialist advice should be sought before embarking on such treatment unless you have particular expertise. Drugs that may be used include methadone, codeine-based drugs, buprenorphine, lofexidine, clonidine and naltrexone.

Untreated heroin withdrawal typically reaches its peak 36–72 hours after the last dose, and symptoms will have subsided substantially after 5 days. Untreated methadone withdrawal is typically over a longer duration with symptoms not subsiding until 10–12 days. The symptoms and signs of opiate withdrawal are shown below.

SYMPTOMS AND SIGNS OF OPIATE WITHDRAWAL

- Sweating.
- Lachrymation and rhinorrhea.
- Yawning.
- Feeling hot and cold.
- Anorexia and abdominal cramps.
- Nausea, vomiting and diarrhoea.
- Tremor.
- Insomnia and restlessness.
- Generalized aches and pains.
- Tachycardia, hypertension.
- Gooseflesh.
- Dilated pupils.
- Increased bowel sounds.

STIMULANT MISUSE

The main stimulants are amphetamines and cocaine. Both groups of drugs result in dependence and withdrawal effects. Acute intoxication results in over-arousal, disinhibition and psychotic symptoms. Withdrawal results in dysphoria, reduced energy and irritability.

COMPLICATIONS OF AMPHETAMINE AND COCAINE MISUSE

Medical
- Cardiovascular: hypertension, arrhythmias.
- Infective: abscesses, hepatitis, septicaemia, HIV.
- Obstetric: reduced foetal growth, miscarriage, placental abruption, premature labour.
- Other: weight loss, dental problems, epilepsy.

Psychiatric
- Anxiety.
- Depression.
- Antisocial behaviours.
- Paranoid psychosis.

Management is largely psychological and social although the use of antidepressant medication may be helpful. Psychotic symptoms need specialist referral. There is no indication for substitute prescribing for cocaine or methylamphetamine. Dexamphetamine may be prescribed for amphetamine abuse to minimize withdrawal and craving. Evidence for its effectiveness is limited, and only GPs with specialist knowledge should consider its use.

Ecstasy (MDMA – methylenedioxymethamphetamine) has both stimulant and hallucinogenic properties. There are rare reports of death due to hyperthermia, cardiac arrhythmias and cerebral haemorrhage. It may be associated with psychotic disorders, and be the precipitating cause in a predisposed individual. Users should be aware of the risks, the need to replace fluid loss and the need to rest during dancing. There is an as yet uncertain risk of long-term neurological damage.

BENZODIAZEPINE MISUSE

Patients dependent on benzodiazepines often do not fit the usual stereotype of the drug misuser. Most doctors are now well aware of the risks of benzodiazepine dependence and have made efforts to discontinue treatment for those patients in whom it is possible. There are some patients, however, for whom the difficulties and risk of discontinuing the benzodiazepine prescriptions outweigh the benefits. For these patients it is important to limit the amount of benzodiazepines prescribed. The main withdrawal symptoms associated with sudden cessation of benzodiazepines are shown in Table 11.3 (overleaf).

Table 11.3. Withdrawal syndrome associated with benzodiazepine use

Anxiety symptoms
Anxiety, sweating, insomnia, headache, tremor, nausea

Disordered perceptions
Feelings of unreality
Abnormal body sensations
Abnormal sensation of movement
Hypersensitivity to stimuli

Major complications
Psychosis
Epileptic seizures

If the decision is made to reduce benzodiazepine use, the current benzodiazepine should be converted to diazepam. Diazepam has the advantage of a relatively long half-life, and it is available in different strength tablets. Table 11.4 shows the appropriate dosages of common benzodiazepines equivalent to 5 mg of diazepam.

Table 11.4. Dosages of common benzodiazepines

Drug	Dose (equivalent to 5 mg diazepam)
Chlordiazepoxide	15 mg
Lorazepam	500 microgram
Oxazepam	15 mg
Temazepam	10 mg
Nitrazepam	5 mg

The principles of the withdrawal regime are as follows:

BENZODIAZEPINE WITHDRAWAL

- Switch to diazepam.
- Withdraw the diazepam by about one-eighth of the daily dose every fortnight.
- At lower doses, the rate can be reduced by about 2.5 mg a fortnight.
- The patient may need to be referred for non-pharmacological anxiety management.
- If insomnia remains a problem, the prescription of a non-benzodiazepine hypnotic for a maximum of 2 weeks may be considered.

PRESCRIBING FOR CONTROLLED DRUGS

The prescription for controlled drugs must state in the prescriber's own handwriting in ink:

- The patient's name and address.
- In the case of a preparation, the form (even when it is implicit in the proprietary name or where only one form is available) and, where appropriate, the strength of the preparation.
- The total quantity of the preparation (the number of dose units) in both words and figures (this does not apply to temazepam).
- The dose.
- Be signed and dated by the prescriber.

A prescription may order a controlled drug to be dispensed by instalments; the amount of the instalments and the intervals to be observed must be specified.

In all cases, a licence is necessary to prescribe cocaine, diamorphine or dipipanone for addicts, except for the treatment of organic disease or injury.

SHARED CARE

The range of specialist services will vary according to the locality. Multidisciplinary working is essential for the appropriate care of substance misusers and should include:

- Specialist medical advice for complex problems.
- Community drug team workers for counselling, keyworkers, needle exchange and so on.
- Social workers for advice on benefits and welfare.
- Pharmacists for daily dispensing.
- Practice nurses for wound care and health education.

WHEN TO REFER

- Presence of severe psychiatric complications, e.g. psychotic symptoms.
- Assessment and management of suicide risk.
- Access to specialist services, e.g. inpatient detoxification services and residential rehabilitation.
- High-risk individuals, e.g. pregnant opiate users.
- Patients requesting opiate replacement therapy.

REFERENCES

Department of Health (1999). *Drug Misuse and Opiate Dependence: Guidelines on Clinical Management*. London Stationery Office, London.

Gerada C, Tighe J (1999). A review of shared care protocols for treatment of problem drug use in England, Scotland and Wales. *British Journal of General Practice* **49**:125–6.

FURTHER READING

Drug Misuse and Dependence (1991). HMSO, London.

Helping Patients who Misuse Drugs (1997). *Drug and Therapeutics Bulletin* **35**:18–22.

WEBSITES

US Homepage for the Center for Education and Drug Abuse Research
www.pih.edu/~cedar
For information, education and publications.

US National Clearing House for Alcohol and Drug Information
www.health.org
For databases, research and on-line courses.

SELF-HELP

Drugline Ltd
9a Brockley Cross, Brockley, London SE4 2AB
Tel: 020 8692 4975

Narcotics Anonymous
Tel: 020 7351 6794/6066
Provides advice, information and counselling.

National Drugs Helpline
Tel: 0800 776600
Provides 24-hour confidential advice including information on local services.

Turning Point
New Loom House, 101 Backchurch Lane, London E1 1LU
Tel: 020 7702 2300

chapter 12

The manic patient

IN THIS CHAPTER

- When to seek specialist assessment.
- Management of mild manic relapse.
- Long-term management of mood stabilizers:
  - guidelines for lithium use,
  - when to stop mood stabilizers.
- Management of depressive episodes in bipolar disorder.

INTRODUCTION

Mania almost invariably occurs as part of a bipolar illness. Thus, even for patients with one or more episodes of mania alone, it is likely that they will have a depressive episode at some stage in the future.

Epidemiology

Table 12.1. Epidemiology of mania
• Lifetime risk 1–1.5%
• Risk factors for onset:
– positive family history
– steroids
• Risk factors for relapse:
– stopping lithium (risk x28 in 3 months after stopping)
– abrupt discontinuation of lithium (less than 14 days)
– life events
• Risk of suicide x12
• Risk of violent death x3

Recognition and diagnosis

Recognition of the patient who is acutely manic does not usually present a difficult, diagnostic dilemma. Such presentations are, however, rare in primary care. Table 12.2 shows the key clinical features of acute mania. The term hypomania describes a lesser degree of mania in which the manic symptoms, although persisting for several days, do not lead to severe social consequences – the symptoms are not accompanied by hallucinations or delusions.

Although the florid presentation of a patient with mania is easy to recognize, it can be difficult to be sure in the early stages of a manic episode whether or not the patient is unwell. It is often the patient's friends or relatives who raise concerns; the patient may not even agree to a consultation. Even when a patient's relatives have indicated a significant change in the patient's mental state, during a brief consultation the patient can appear to be well and give rational and reasonable explanations for their relatives' concerns. It is important to remember that unless extremely unwell, patients with mania can keep control of their symptoms during a brief

Table 12.2. Clinical features of mania

Mood: infectious cheerfulness, euphoria, irritability

Behaviour: distractible, over-spending, promiscuity

Self-esteem: self-confidence, grandiose, over-optimistic ideas, reckless decisions

Energy: overactive, decreased sleep

Speech: loud, rapid, pressure, flight of ideas, rhymes, puns, inappropriate familiarity

Psychotic symptoms: delusional beliefs about wealth, special powers, hallucinations

Insight: often impaired

interview. Mania can cause considerable social disruption to the patient's life with consequences lasting long after the episode of illness, because of over-spending, promiscuity and irritability and rudeness. Patients with mania often have a feeling of wellbeing and little, if any, recognition of illness. Hence it is important that if relatives raise what are considered to be reasonable concerns, steps are taken to protect the patient, including early consideration of an assessment under the Mental Health Act.

A second important point when considering a diagnosis of mania is the presence of irritability rather than euphoria as the key symptom of mood in mania. The patient may come across simply as abrupt and boorish rather than euphoric. Manic patients often have an uncanny knack of picking out personal features or habits about which you might be sensitive, such as being overweight or hair loss, and then commenting inappropriately on them. At a more extreme level, manic patients can be extremely hostile and threatening. In such cases, confrontations should be avoided (see Chapter 15) and swift recourse to the police and an assessment under the Mental Health Act needs to be made.

There is an increased risk of co-morbid substance/alcohol misuse (x6) amongst patients with a bipolar disorder.

Cyclothymia

Cyclothymia is the term used to describe recurrent mood swings that do not meet diagnostic criteria for mania or depression. It describes lability of mood that is more a feature of the patient's personality rather than an illness.

MANAGEMENT IN PRIMARY CARE

✓ Acute mania.
✓ Manic relapse.
✓ Long-term prophylaxis.
✓ Depressive relapse.

Acute mania

The management of the acute phase of a manic episode is largely under-taken by the specialist mental health services. Treatment often requires inpatient care and the use of mood stabilizers, neuroleptic and sedative drugs. The GP is most likely to be directly involved in three phases:

- The recognition and early management of a manic relapse.
- The long-term prophylaxis.
- The recognition and management of a depressive relapse.

Recognition and management of a manic relapse

The early stages of a manic relapse are often perceived as welcome by the patient. The patient has a sense of well-being and a feeling of 'can do'. This is accompanied by increased energy and a reduced need to sleep. In this phase, patients are often extremely productive. Sadly, however, such episodes can lead swiftly to the more destructive phase of mania as noted above. It is important, therefore, that the patient is taught to recognize early symptoms and seek medical advice.

It can be difficult to judge whether a patient's sense of well-being is normal mood or the early stages of mania. Patients may learn to recognize their own symptoms which herald relapse (a 'relapse signature'). A common and easy symptom to measure and evaluate is the reduced need for sleep. Although everyone can have the occasional disturbed night, the reduced need for sleep in mania is accompanied by a feeling of wanting to get up and do activities. The patient who unusually wakes at 4 or 5 am and gets up to start working should be recognized as needing treatment.

Although treatment should involve a referral to the specialist mental health services for assessment and help, the GP may have a role in the treatment of a mild relapse.

WHAT TO DO IN MILD MANIC RELAPSE

- Check the level of mood stabilizer.
- Give benzodiazepine to aid sleep.
- Consider a sedative antipsychotic:
  - chlorpromazine,
  - haloperidol.
- Advise the patient:
  - not to drive,
  - not to work,
  - to avoid important business/social decisions.
- Involve the family if possible.
- Keep the patient under close review.

Long-term prophylaxis

Many patients with a bipolar disorder will be on long term-mood stabilizers. The drug which has been available for the longest and is most widely prescribed is lithium. Lithium is usually started by a specialist, but once the patient has stabilized on the drug, long-term management often returns to primary care. Although there has been some discussion about the effectiveness of lithium, it is generally agreed that the drug reduces the frequency of manic relapses by about half. Lithium is a drug that needs to be taken in the long term and at least for a minimum of 2 years. There is evidence that early discontinuation of lithium brings forward a manic episode.

Lithium has a fairly narrow therapeutic window and hence needs careful monitoring to be prescribed safely and effectively. Before starting lithium, thyroid and renal functions need to be checked. Serum creatinine, if normal, is adequate evidence of satisfactory renal function. In patients with a history of cardiac abnormality an ECG should be recorded. The key points in the management of lithium are set out below.

MANAGEMENT OF LITHIUM

- Women of child-bearing age should be using reliable contraception.
- Lithium should be prescribed in a once daily night-time dose.
- Lithium should be prescribed by brand name.
- Serum lithium levels should be taken 10–14 hours after the last dose.
- Lithium levels should be checked every 3–6 months.
- Annual measurement of thyroid function, serum creatinine, serum calcium.
- For prophylaxis in patients with bipolar disorder, serum levels of 0.5–1.0 mmol/l should be maintained.
- Patients should be informed of the benefits and risks and told to stop lithium immediately, and seek medical advice, if they have diarrhoea and/or vomiting.

(Drugs and Therapeutics Bulletin, 1999)

Lithium is teratogenic and hence women of child-bearing age should be advised to use reliable contraception. Lithium's teratogenic effects are most frequent in the first trimester. Lithium should be prescribed by its generic name because of differences in bio-availability between the different products.

The side-effects of lithium are set out in Table 12.3.

If side-effects are troublesome, reducing the dose may relieve the side-effects but still maintain adequate prophylaxis. The most bothersome side-

---

Table 12.3. Lithium side-effects

- Gastrointestinal:
  - gastrointestinal upset (1)
  - weight gain (3)
  - dry mouth and metallic taste (5)
- Renal:
  - thirst and polyuria (2)
- Neurological:
  - fatigue and sleepiness (4)
  - memory impairment and mental slowness
  - fine tremor
- Endocrine:
  - hypothyroidism
  - hypoparathyroidism
- Dermatological:
  - exacerbate psoriasis

(n) = order of frequency of occurrence (Gitalin *et al.*, 1989).

---

effects relate to weight gain and reduced mental acuity (Gitalin *et al.*, 1989).

The precise drug level to achieve prophylaxis with the minimum of side-effects will vary between patients. Some authors indicate that doses at the lower end of the therapeutic range, e.g. 0.5–0.8 mmol/l, are adequate, although patients with higher levels (0.8–1.0 mmol/l) may be at less risk of relapse. The precise level needed for each individual patient will vary, and it is important to balance prophylaxis against side-effects which are clearly less at the reduced doses.

Lithium can, of course, be toxic; toxicity usually occurs when the serum lithium concentration is more than 1.5 mmol/l. Risky times are when the patient is dehydrated, e.g. through gastroenteritis or a hot climate. Co-prescription of drugs which reduce lithium excretion, e.g. thiazide diuretics and NSAIDs, can increase lithium levels. Clinical features to identify lithium toxicity are set out below.

LITHIUM TOXICITY

- Ataxia.
- Coarse tremor.
- Muscle twitching and increased muscle tone.
- Slurred speech.
- Confusion.

When to stop mood stabilizers

The decision to stop mood stabilizers depends on the risk of relapse compared to the problems of continuing with medication. This is a decision best taken by the patient when fully appraised of the facts. The individual decision can be greatly helped by a life chart (Figure 12.1). This life chart helped the patient with the decision to stay on lithium. In another patient such a chart may show lithium to have little prophylactic value.

Lithium should not be stopped abruptly, but over a minimum of 1 month. The risk of relapse is high in the early weeks following discontinuation.

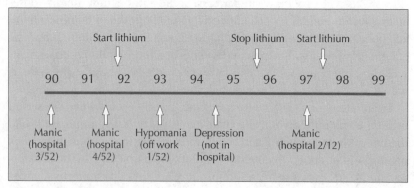

Figure 12.1. Life chart.

Psychological advice

There is some evidence that maintaining a regular routine protects against relapse. Similarly, disruptions to such a routine, e.g. shift work, jet lag and major social changes, are times of increased risk. Although patients cannot lead lives cocooned against social stresses, awareness of the importance of regular routines and extra vigilance if these are broken is sensible advice.

Management of depressive relapse

The management of depressive episodes in patients with bipolar disorder presents a difficulty. This is because of the risk of any antidepressant medication chosen precipitating a manic episode. Hence it is often wise to seek a specialist opinion if a depressive episode persists. Optimizing the doses of mood stabilizing medication is often the first step. There is little evidence that any of the antidepressants are either worse or better at causing a manic switch. The principle to follow is to use lower doses of antidepressant medication, and also to avoid drugs with a long half-life, such as fluoxetine. The use of psychological interventions to treat the depression should clearly be considered, not only would this be likely to avoid the risk of a manic switch, but also the patient might then be equipped with skills to handle depressive episodes in the future.

WHEN TO REFER

- All patients presenting with clear symptoms of mania.
- Patients engaging in harmful behaviours – early assessment under the Mental Health Act should be arranged if they are unwilling to seek specialist help.
- Patients with persisting depressive symptoms in the context of bipolar disorder.
- Patients on long-term mood stabilizers who wish to have specialist advice about the continuing need for treatment.

TREATMENT IN SECONDARY CARE

Patients with bipolar affective disorders have a chronic illness. Many are disabled by their recurring symptoms, and others have to cope with the aftermath of manic behaviours which makes their lives difficult, even when symptom free. Such patients, therefore, are often under regular follow up by psychiatric teams. A range of support, pharmacological, emotional and practical, may be required.

In addition to lithium, there are two other mood-stabilizing drugs licensed for the management of bipolar affective disorders, and two drugs which are being used for more resistant cases, but for which there is much less evidence. All these drugs are anticonvulsants.

Carbamazepine

Carbamazepine has long been used as a second-line treatment for patients refractory or intolerant to lithium. There is evidence that it is as effective as lithium and it can be considered as a first-line mood stabilizer. In particular, there is some evidence that carbamazepine may be more effective than lithium in patients with frequent mood swings. Carbamazepine may be used either on its own, or in combination with lithium. The usual dose is in the range of 400–1600 mg daily given in divided doses. There is no clear prophylactic dose range as with lithium, but a target serum level of 8–12 mg/l has been recommended.

CARBAMAZEPINE: SIDE-EFFECTS

- Worse at the start of treatment.
- Drowsiness.
- Dizziness.
- Diplopia.
- Nausea.
- Erythematous rash (5–10%).
- Weight gain (8%).
- Agranulocytosis (1 in 20 000).

Carbamazepine increases the metabolism of other drugs, including TCAs, benzodiazepines, haloperidol, oral contraceptives, thyroxine and other anticonvulsants. The drug also induces its own metabolism and hence plasma carbamazepine levels may fall after the first few weeks of treatment.

Sodium valproate
There is evidence that sodium valproate is effective in the acute management of mania, but there are no controlled trials of its efficacy in the prophylaxis of bipolar disorder.

Gabapentin and lamotrigine
Gabapentin and lamotrigine are two other anticonvulsants that are being used experimentally in the treatment of mania.

PSYCHOLOGICAL TREATMENTS

There is some evidence that the combination of psychological treatments together with drug treatments both improves compliance with the drug treatment, and also improves patient outcome. It is likely that the therapeutic gains result from enhancing the patients' understanding of their illness and the need for prophylactic medication, together with helping them to overcome the difficulties caused by the recurrent, and as noted above, often destructive nature of the disorder.

REFERENCES

Drugs and Therapeutics Bulletin (1999). Using lithium safely. *Drugs and Therapeutics Bulletin* **37**:22–4

Gitalin NJ , Cochrane SD, Jamison KR (1989). Maintenance lithium treatment side effects and compliance. *Journal of Clinical Psychiatry* **50**:127–31.

FURTHER READING

Jamison K (1997). *An Unquiet Mind.* Vintage Books, London.
A personal account of bipolar disorder from an international expert in the field.

WEBSITE

Mental Health Net – Bipolar Disorder
www.mentalhelth.net
Useful fact sheets about bipolar and other disorders.

SELF-HELP

Manic Depression Fellowship
8–10 High Street, Kingston-on-Thames KT1 1EY
Tel: 020 8974 6550
Provides support, advice and information for people with manic depression, their families, friends and carers.

Manic Depression Fellowship (Scotland)
7 Woodside Crescent, Glasgow G37 UL
Tel: 0141 331 0344
Provides support, advice and information for people with manic depression, their families, friends and carers.

Manic Depression Fellowship (Wales)
Belmont, St Cadoc's Hospital, Caerleon, Newport NP6 1XQ
Tel: 01633 430430
Provides support, advice and information for people with manic depression, their families, friends and carers.

chapter 13

The patient with a personality disorder

IN THIS CHAPTER

- What is a personality disorder?
  - antisocial personality disorder,
  - borderline personality disorder.
- Managing personality disorders in primary care:
  - limit setting,
  - drug treatments.
- When secondary care should be involved.

INTRODUCTION

Patients with personality disorders can be amongst the most difficult patients to treat in general practice. All GPs will have had the experience of referring a patient to a specialist psychiatric service only to have them assessed as having a personality disorder, with no treatable psychiatric diagnosis, and sent back to primary care. The GP is then left with the unenviable task of attempting to manage a patient who is often very demanding and also disabled by their symptoms.

It has been suggested that the term 'personality disorder' should no longer be used in that it is a pejorative term with little value in determining treatment or prognosis. However, it is likely that the term will remain in use for those patients without clear psychiatric diagnoses who continue to have personal and social difficulties that can not easily be summed up in any other succinct way.

If the term personality disorder is to have any validity, it should be restricted for patients with the following features:

WHAT IS A PERSONALITY DISORDER?

- An enduring , abnormal pattern of attitudes and behaviour involving several areas of functioning including cognition, affect, interpersonal functioning and impulse control.
- The abnormal pattern is long-standing, often dating back to early adulthood and not limited to episodes of mental illness.
- The abnormal pattern leads to clinically significant distress (to self or others), or impairment in social, occupational or other important areas of functioning.

EPIDEMIOLOGY

Early studies indicate that GPs diagnose personality disorders in about 5% of their patients. The most thorough study of personality disorders done in UK primary care, using a standardized interview, found that a startling 34% had a personality disorder (Casey *et al.*, 1984). The most common associations were with diagnoses of anxiety states and alcohol abuse. Although there is probable agreement at the severe end of the personality disorder spectrum, there is as little consensus, within the research literature, as in clinical practice, as to definitions of mild/moderate disorder.

Patients with a personality disorder are at increased risk of suicide and premature death. The more severe the symptoms and behaviours, the worse the long-term outcome. If personality disordered patients survive, they often seem to improve with age and maturity. Poor prognostic factors include parental brutality and concurrent substance misuse.

DIAGNOSIS

The diagnosis of a personality disorder may be better made by a GP than by a psychiatrist. The GP is often in a better position to distinguish between transient and enduring patterns of behaviour. GPs are unlikely, however, to be called upon to make a diagnosis as to the specific type of personality disorder. The ICD-10 currently lists eight types: paranoid, schizoid, dissocial, emotionally unstable (impulsive and borderline types), histrionic, anankastic, anxious (avoidant) and dependent. It is often more helpful to consider the presence or absence of specific personality traits, e.g. impulsivity and low self-esteem, rather than to try to force a patient's characteristics into a particular personality type. The two personality diagnoses with the most validity, and about which most has been written, are antisocial and borderline, hence these will be discussed in more detail.

Antisocial personality disorder

DIAGNOSTIC CRITERIA

There is a pervasive pattern of disregard for, and violation of, the rights of others occurring since the age of 15 years as indicated by three or more of the following:

- Failure to conform to social norms with respect to lawful behaviours as indicated by repeatedly performing illegal acts.
- Deceitfulness, repeated lying, use of alias.
- Impulsivity.
- Irritability and aggressiveness as indicated by repeated physical fights or assaults.
- Reckless disregard for safety of self or others.
- Consistent irresponsibility indicated by repeated failure to sustain consistent work or honour financial obligations.
- Lack of remorse.

(DSM-IV, 1994)

The terminology around antisocial personality disorder is confusing. DSM-IV uses the term 'antisocial personality disorder', the ICD-10 uses the term 'dissocial personality disorder', whereas the Mental Health Act 1983 uses the term 'psychopathic personality disorder'.

In essence, the behaviour of people with an antisocial personality disorder is greatly at odds with the prevailing social norms. There is a callous unconcern for the feelings of others. The individual will have great difficulty in sustaining any long-term relationships, although will often have no problem in establishing new relationships. There is a low threshold for the tolerance of frustration, which can lead to aggression and, ultimately, serious violence. Legal restrictions and punishment do not seem to have any specific deterrent effect, as individuals experience neither guilt nor remorse for their actions. To further compound matters, individuals are poor and unreliable historians. Joint working between health services, social services and the criminal justice system is required for best management of such individuals.

There is a continuing political debate as to whether individuals with an antisocial personality are mad, bad or both, to what extent they are responsible for their actions and whether they can be treated in whole or part.

Borderline personality disorder

DIAGNOSTIC CRITERIA

A pervasive pattern of instability of interpersonal relationships, self-image, affect and marked impulsivity indicated by five or more of the following:

- Frantic efforts to avoid real or imagined abandonment.
- A pattern of unstable and intense interpersonal relationships.
- Unstable self-image.
- Impulsivity in at least two areas which are potentially self-damaging, e.g. spending, sex, substance abuse, reckless driving and binge eating.

- Recurrent suicidal behaviour gestures or threats.
- Affective instability due to marked reactivity of mood.
- Chronic feelings of emptiness.
- Inappropriate intense anger or difficulty controlling anger.
- Transient stress-related paranoid ideation.

(DSM-IV, 1994)

The term 'borderline personality disorder' is probably the most useful clinically of the personality disorders in that it defines a recognizable group of patients who frequently present for help. The term 'borderline' begs the question, borderline to what? It probably refers to the borderline between neurotic and psychotic disorders in that such patients can develop transient psychotic symptoms when under stress. Other salient features are unstable mood, unstable relationships and unstable identity. Many borderline patients have been sexually abused. Specific treatment programmes have been developed to help such patients.

MANAGEMENT IN PRIMARY CARE

The management of patients with personality disorders should focus on the management of particular symptoms or behaviours rather than attempting a global personality change. Personality disorders should be seen as a chronic disorder with fluctuating symptoms. The aim of treatment is to optimize function and not cure. Patients with personality disorders may develop a clear-cut psychiatric illness, such as a depressive disorder, which should be treated as appropriate, although evidence suggests that treatments are less effective in the presence of a personality disorder.

It is important that the GP is very clear about the limits of treatment. Patients need to be encouraged to take responsibility for their actions and not blame them on their symptoms or the failures of others.

Managing personality disorders in primary care

- Is there a specific problem or symptom I can help resolve?
- Is there a co-morbid psychiatric disorder which merits treatment or referral?
- Would it be helpful to set aside regular appointments to avoid reinforcing maladaptive behaviours in a crisis? The principles of such appointments being to engage, contain and maintain.
- Keep consultations to time.
- Do not accept responsibility for the patient's actions and/or threats.

Drug treatments may have a role in the management of symptoms in personality disorders. Such treatments should always be considered as an empirical trial without undue hopes being raised, and stopping the treatments if they are ineffective. Table 13.1 gives an indication of symptoms and drugs that might be appropriate. Benzodiazepines should be avoided, both because of the risk of dependency and abuse, and also because of the small risk of precipitating a rage reaction.

Table 13.1. Drug treatment for symptoms in patients with personality disorder

Symptom	Drug
Labile mood	SSRI or related antidepressant
Anger	Low-dose neuroleptic
Impulsive behaviour (bingeing, self-harming)	SSRI (high dose) Consider adding low-dose neuroleptic
Suspicious, paranoid	Low-dose neuroleptic

Another consideration is whether to agree in advance a crisis plan with the patient. What should be done when the patient feels angry/over-whelmed/suicidal?

WHEN TO REFER

✓ Threatening patients.
✓ Anger management.
✓ Deliberate self-harm.
✓ Co-morbidity.

Threatening patients

Patients with personality disorders may make excessive demands on their GP in terms of time, night calls, or requests for repeat or increased medications, occasionally with an air of menace. This can also be in combination with a shifting of responsibility for their actions. In extreme cases, it can be viewed as the GP being blamed by the patient for any subsequent acts of deliberate self-harm or violence. When confronted with such behaviour, or threats of such behaviour, this should act as a trigger for a specialist referral for an assessment of the diagnosis, level of risk and the formulation of an appropriate management plan (see Chapter 15).

Anger management

Some young men are prone to impulsive, angry outbursts, which can lead to assaultative behaviour and damage to property. In recent times, a trend has started where these young men, following arrest for assault, have been advised by their solicitor to go to their GP seeking help with their temper or requesting 'anger management'. There is some limited evidence that anger management groups are of help to some. Such treatment emphasizes the need for individuals to accept responsibility for their own actions and not to shift the blame on to others. Anger management is, however, not available in all areas.

Repeat deliberate self-harm

Impulsive overdoses, wrist cutting and other acts of deliberate self-harm, may result in attendance at the local accident and emergency department with subsequent hospitalization until the patient is medically fit to be discharged. It is not unusual for such patients to discharge themselves against medical advice. The individuals are at increased risk of further self-harming behaviour and of completed suicide (see Chapter 15).

Co-morbidity

Patients are rarely referred to secondary care with a primary diagnosis of personality disorder. There is a high prevalence of co-morbid disorders, such as depression, anxiety, somatization and alcohol/drug misuse. Such disorders often respond poorly to simple treatments. It may also be helpful when managing a patient with a personality disorder to make use of specialist care for assistance in managing the co-morbid conditions of alcohol misuse and drug-related problems. Secondary care can also provide assistance in the assessment and management of risk.

WHAT TO EXPECT FROM SECONDARY CARE

As a group of disorders, the personality disorders provide the professional worker with a singular challenge with regard to their on-going management. This is because, as Casey (1998) reminds us, 'the disorders are almost impossible to define, may have no actual symptoms, are of unknown cause, and also may lack any specific treatment and barely fit into the concept of medical disease'.

Secondary care has no magic pill or treatment to offer patients with personality disorders; however, all services should be able to offer:

- An assessment resulting in a diagnosis and list of patient problems.
- An assessment of risk to both self and others.

If secondary care accepts such patients, the aims of involvement are:

- Engagement.
- Containment.
- Maintenance.
- Harm reduction.

Local services will vary, but the following may be available:

- Specialist psychological treatment for patients who have been sexually abused.
- Specialist psychological treatment to facilitate engagement and treatment of patients with borderline personality disorder.
- Anger management groups.

A CMHT may allocate a keyworker to the more disturbed of such patients to help limit maladaptive behaviours. The skills such a practitioner needs to offer are:

- *Experience:* the ability to 'hold one's nerve' when faced with threats or the prospect of deliberate self-harm.
- *Continuity:* in working with personality disordered patients it may take a long time to form a bond of trust. A patient who has had repeated changes of keyworker may regard the attempt by the worker to develop a therapeutic relationship as being built up to be knocked down if the worker leaves.
- *Acceptance of the limitations of treatment:* no intervention will quickly reduce ingrained patterns of maladaptive coping strategies.
- *Provision of open and honest feedback:* patients need to be made aware of the effect of their behaviours on others, but in an exploratory and problem-solving way rather than in a judgemental and critical way.
- *Liaison with other agencies:* there will be occasions when it is essential to work with other agencies, such as the local authority social services department if child protection issues arise, or the criminal justice system.
- *Team working:* this group of patients can evoke strong personal reactions, often causing 'splitting' between team members as to what would be the most effective intervention or treatment rationale.

It is not true that nothing can be done for patients with personality disorders. Patients may not be 'cured', but they can be supported through crises and helped to lead more normal lives. Patients must, for the most part, take responsibility for their actions and be prepared to engage with professionals. Inpatient psychiatric care is generally unhelpful and counterproductive, and can lead to escalation in self-harming and destructive behaviours.

CASE STUDY: TOM

Tom turns up towards the end of Dr Jones's evening surgery frantically requesting benzodiazepines to calm him down as he is going through a particularly stressful time. Tom registered at the practice about 6 months ago, having been allocated a single person's flat by a local housing association. Tom has consulted as an emergency on three occasions seeing different partners during that time. Dr Jones briefly scans the correspondence in the notes.

Tom is the eldest of four siblings, his mother never married, the children's fathers being three different men. Between the ages of 3 and 6 years, Tom was in foster care and during that time was placed with five families and spent 10 months in residential care. As Tom's mother adopted a more settled lifestyle, he returned to the family home with her new partner and his younger brother and sister. His mother's new partner had convictions for violence and drug offences, and did not get on well with Tom; eventually all four children were taken into care.

From about the age of 12 years, Tom's life became a succession of transfers between foster families and childrens' homes. He frequently truanted from school and developed a growing antipathy to authority figures. This led to him having repeated confrontations with school teachers, foster parents, social workers and the police. By the age of 14 years he was regularly drinking, inhaling solvents, smoking cannabis and using amphetamines. It was after a drug binge that Tom first cut his wrists. Tom was offered a referral to an adolescent unit and a drugs counsellor, but he did not attend.

Tom absconded from care and went to live in London. He cut his wrists intermittently and, on one occasion, was arrested on section 136 of the Mental Health Act 1983 after saying that he was going to jump off a multi-storey car park. He was admitted to hospital for assessment, but was not thought to be mentally ill and took his own discharge. Tom declined any follow up, or help with his drug and alcohol use.

Tom returned to his home town and was subsequently arrested and convicted of possession of a weapon and threatening behaviour. A condition of his probation order was that he needed supervision and a permanent address. It was at this time that Tom moved into a hostel and seemed to embark upon a more settled period of his life. Tom seemed to benefit from the order and structure that the hostel offered: his drinking and drug use was curtailed, but he still had occasional binges. He would still self-harm by wrist cutting a couple of times a year without any clear precipitant. A previous GP who covered the hostel commenced Tom on fluoxetine and saw Tom weekly when he attended the hostel to run a clinic. During this time, Tom's mood and general outlook on life became more positive, his self-harming diminished and he began to attend a local MIND day centre. The day centre offered Tom a supportive environment and he began to make friends and get practical help in managing his benefits.

Tom was allocated a single person's flat and moved in about 6 months ago. He continued to attend the day centre, but missed the companionship of the other hostel residents in the evening. He started going to the pub and frequently drank to excess.

It is not clear what has caused the current crisis – Tom says the neighbours at his flat are 'doing his head in'. Dr Jones sees Tom and prescribes trifluoperazine 5 mg at night to help reduce his anxiety. He asks Tom to make a regular appointment for the next week. To Dr Jones's surprise Tom keeps the appointment and Dr Jones writes to the social worker at the local CMHT to see if increased social support could be provided.

Lessons from the case study

- Personality disorder has a fluctuating course.
- Regular, structured involvement can be helpful.
- Judicious prescribing may assist.
- Goals are improved functioning, not cure.
- Non-judgemental interventions.

REFERENCES

Casey PR, Tyrer PJ, Dillon S (1984). The diagnostic status of patients with conspicuous psychiatric morbidity in primary care. *Psychological Medicine* **14**:673–81.

Casey P (1998). *Personality Disorders in Seminars in General Psychiatry*, vol. 2 (eds. Stein and Wilkinson). Royal College of Psychiatrists: Gaskell, London.

DSM-IV (1994). *Diagnositc and Statistical Manual of Mental Disorders*. American Psychiatric Association, Washington DC.

WEBSITES

Borderline Personality Disorder Centre
www.BDPCentral.com
Provides information regarding borderline personality disorder. This website is American and may use terminology that is unfamiliar to the British reader.

SELF-HELP

There are no specific groups catering for people with personality disorders – any self-help comes from the associated co-morbid presentations. Self-help may be obtained by attendance at voluntary groups or day centres run by organizations, such as Alcoholics Anonymous, MIND and the National Schizophrenia Fellowship (NSF).

chapter 14

The bereaved patient

IN THIS CHAPTER

- What is 'normal bereavement'?
- Risk factors for the likelihood of a complicated grief reaction.
- Appropriate interventions following bereavement.
- Coping with cot death.

INTRODUCTION

Bereavement is a common and distressing experience. For the vast majority of patients, common humanity suggests sympathy, empathy and understanding are required. There may be a temptation to do more: prescribe medication, or refer on to specialized help. However, this is only required in a minority of cases. Most people manage to make the emotional and social adjustments required following bereavement without the need for mental health interventions.

RECOGNITION AND DIAGNOSIS

Normal bereavement

Whilst there are stages in grieving and bereavement, it is certainly not a 'one model fits all'. There are considerable cultural variations and individual differences. Progression through stages may not occur in a linear fashion. Many patients comment that 'you don't get over bereavement, you learn to live with it', and report that many years after a loss there can be pangs of sorrow and tears. However, it is uncommon for the aching distress of bereavement to be maintained.

At the time of death, or when news is first broken, there is often a reaction of acute distress, which may be followed quickly by a feeling of being stunned and feeling as though the death has not happened. People often describe feeling emotionally numb. There can also be an internal battle between wanting to cry out and wail, and a need to stay in control. There is also often anger, which may be directed at people who had been caring for the dead person or members of the close family. These reactions are usually regretted later.

The initial stage is followed by severe distress, grief and yearning for the dead person. This is commonly interspersed with periods of apathy. Such variability of emotion can be confusing for the bereaved and carers. Any reminder of the loss can trigger the pangs of grieving. The intensity of these feelings can often lead to sleep disturbance, appetite disturbance and concentration difficulties. This may be accompanied by some minor memory disturbance. Recurrent recollections of the events leading up to the loss are common. There may also be self-blaming for the death or anger with others. Within families this can sometimes lead to estrangement. There can be feelings of guilt. This may be associated with feeling understandable relief after a long or painful illness, or from having feelings of anger towards the dead person, or feeling that things have been left unsaid. It is commonly reported by the bereaved that they mistakenly think that they have seen the lost person, and there can be vivid dreams or hypnogogic hallucinations.

With time, resolution occurs and the acute pain of bereavement begins to fade, along with feelings of depression. There is no reliable guide to the length of time bereavement lasts; however, many individuals report their feelings of hopelessness and despair reach a peak between 4–6 weeks after the death. There may still be episodes of grief triggered by any one of a number of cues, many months or years after the bereavement. The bereaved and others can find this embarrassing.

Following bereavement there is a greater likelihood of physical illness. There is also increased mortality in the bereaved, especially the older widower.

ABNORMAL OR COMPLICATED GRIEF REACTIONS

Patients will present in a number of ways which may lead the GP to consider an abnormal grief reaction. The patient may have a good insight into the central cause of their distress, or they may present with what they believe is a medical or psychological problem, completely unaware of the role bereavement is playing.

TYPES OF COMPLICATED GRIEF REACTIONS

- Delayed/inhibited grief.
- Chronic grief.
- Excessive care giving.
- Conflict in grief.
- Identification reaction.

- Delayed/inhibited grief: this may occur when, after many months or even years, the expression of distress comes to the fore. Patients may not recognize the bereavement as linked to the distress. Particular circumstances of the bereavement, e.g. looking after the needs of others or fears of losing control, are often thought to be associated with the phenomena.
- Chronic grief: the phase of severe grief persists and individuals may remain overly focussed and preoccupied with the loss. Feelings of depression and withdrawal from others are common.
- Excessive care giving: this may occur as a way of trying to reduce feelings of distress and, in some psychological formulations, is seen as a 'replacement' for care the bereaved individual feels they have not received.
- Conflict in grief: anger and guilt are common reactions following bereavement. If there had been strains in the relationship with the deceased, or a re-awakening of traumatic material in the bereaved, this may lead to complicated bereavement reactions.
- Identification reaction: the bereaved may take on some of the mannerisms or interests of the deceased. There can also be preoccupation with similar symptoms to those experienced by the deceased.

A number of clues which may suggest a complicated grief reaction and the risk factors increasing the likelihood of a complicated grief reactions are outlined below.

CLUES TO COMPLICATED BEREAVEMENT REACTIONS

- Intense and easily triggered grief still regularly present after 6 months.
- Unwillingness to deal with the material possessions of the deceased, or maintenance of a 'shrine' in the house.
- Recurrent symptoms like those experienced by the deceased, hypochondriacal preoccupation.
- Radical changes in lifestyle; exclusion of family and friends.
- Marked and persistent anger.
- Persistent subclinical depression, anxiety or state of elation.
- Imitation of the deceased's characteristics or interests.
- Self-harm, parasuicidal behaviours.
- Intense 'anniversary' distress.
- Avoidance of grieving rituals, or little evidence of normal grieving.

RISK FACTORS INCREASING THE LIKELIHOOD OF A COMPLICATED GRIEF REACTION

Vulnerability of the person
- Past psychiatric history, suicide attempts, low self-esteem.
- Poor social support network, absent family or family difficulties.
- In childhood, relationship difficulties with their parents.
- Ambivalence about their relationship with the deceased.
- Dependent relationship with the deceased.

Nature of the death
- Loss of spouse or child.
- Loss of parent for the child or adolescent.
- Suicide, murder.
- Traumatic death.
- Sudden, unexpected death.

MANAGEMENT IN PRIMARY CARE

The GP and members of the primary health care team are often in a position to offer support and care to the bereaved. There may be a temptation to step back at the time of bereavement because it is felt there is little to be done by a GP. Kindness, emotional support and being able to communicate information in a calm and gentle manner are remembered by patients. Care should be taken to make sure practical help is readily at hand.

Being with a patient and allowing them to grieve rather than eloquent words of comfort are important. Relatives or carers should be encouraged to allow the bereaved to talk and cry, and be told that the bereaved person may need to go over the same things many times. Reassuring people there is no one right way to grieve can be helpful as well. In Western societies, there is a widely-held view that 'letting go' of emotions can lead to a breakdown or madness. Giving people permission to grieve is sometimes important, together with reassurance that expressing such emotions will not lead to loss of control. Bereavement can also result in people facing their own mortality and vulnerability, which can result in symptoms of anxiety.

Seeing a patient to keep an eye on their bereavement and providing time and support is all that is required for the majority of bereaved patients. However, for complicated bereavement reactions or where the GP has identified particular risk factors, additional interventions are necessary. Few GPs will have the time available for specific therapy work with an individual with a complicated bereavement reaction, and in most cases onward referral will be required. It is common for physical symptoms to be part of a complicated bereavement reaction, and before onward referral takes place it is important to exclude physical disease.

INTERVENTIONS: COMPLICATED BEREAVEMENT REACTIONS

- Give the patient permission to grieve.
- Always check out their physical symptoms.
- Check for suicidal ideation.
- Consider an antidepressant and the brief use of hypnotics or anxiolytics.

COT DEATHS

In 1998, there were 344 cot deaths in the UK. This is a rate of 0.46 per 1000 live births per year; 92% occur in children under 6 months. In a group practice of two to three doctors, you might expect to see one case every 4–6 years.

A useful article by Fintan Coyle (1999) sets out the role of the GP:

Contact the family

As soon as you hear of the baby's death, contact the family to express sympathy, by telephone first and then a home visit if possible. Always use the baby's name. Listening is more important than talking. You can not make bereaved families feel better, but do not underestimate the value of your support. Compassion, not cold professionalism, is needed.

Coroner's role

Explain the coroner's duty, the possibility of an inquest and that the parents or relatives may be asked to formally identify the body. The parents will be asked to make a statement to the coroner's office or police. Bedding may be taken for examination to help establish the cause of death.

Cuddling

Allow parents time with their baby for as long as they wish after the death is confirmed.

Call helplines

The Foundation for the Study of Infant Death (FSID) has a 24-hour helpline (020 7235 1721) which offers immediate support and practical advice for families. It also offers free phonecards so parents do not pay for calls.

Ceasing lactation

Give advice on suppression of lactation: wear a firm bra, reduce the intake of fluid, drink only when thirsty and do not rub or massage the nipples. Medications may be needed.

Consider sedatives

Many parents later regret taking anxiolytics or antidepressants which impede decision making and delay grieving. Most just want help with sleep.

Children

Reassure parents that older children are not at risk. Twin babies carry extra risk of cot death – a surviving twin may need hospitalization for observation. Siblings need to be involved, reassured, understood and noticed. Their commonest anxieties are:

'Did I cause it?'
'Will I die too?'
'Who cares for me now?'

When there is a belief in an afterlife, it is important that children understand that it is not the dead body that goes to heaven, but that the parents believe that the dead child's soul is in heaven. Siblings will usually benefit from being included in the funeral and viewing rituals, but they need proper preparation and explanation beforehand. They need to understand the permanence of death (Black, 1998).

Criticism
Anger, sometimes directed towards the GP, guilt and self-blame, especially on the part of the mother, are common grief reactions for which you should be prepared. Parents who have lost a baby often change doctors – do not take it personally.

Coming to terms
Advise parents of likely grief reactions, such as aching arms (due to a longing to hold the baby), hearing the baby cry, distressing dreams, and strong positive or negative sexual feelings, and reassure them that these and other symptoms, such as loss of appetite and sleeplessness, are normal and temporary.

Counselling
Some patients will ask for, or need, counselling; be aware of the local options. FSID offers a befriending scheme.

Cause of death
Make sure the coroner informs you of the initial and final post-mortem findings, and consult with the pathologist if any clarification is needed. Then arrange a subsequent meeting with the parents to discuss the cause of death.

Consultant opinion
Offer parents a later interview with a consultant paediatrician both for themselves and the siblings. An independent opinion is mutually beneficial to the parents and GP – restoring parental confidence in the primary care team and sharing some of the counselling, particularly concerning future children.

Coping in the future
The parents will need extra attention and support with their subsequent children from their obstetrician, paediatrician, GP and health visitor.

Coping yourself
Who will support you through this period? The FSID's 24-hour helpline supports professionals as well as families.

WHEN TO REFER

- If the patient has a past history of serious mental illness or there is serious concern about their mental health, refer them to the CMHT.
- In complicated grief reactions that have not responded to simple measures, consider referral to:
  - in-house counselling,
  - a specialist bereavement therapy service,
  - a voluntary counselling organization.

WHAT TO EXPECT FROM SECONDARY CARE

There is little research evidence to favour one type of intervention over another, or indeed strong research evidence regarding the efficacy of interventions (Kato and Mann, 1999). However, the majority of research in this area has been of poor quality and few, if any, conclusions can be drawn. Most therapy involves an initial assessment, followed by regular weekly or bi-weekly individual or group sessions. Time is spent initially talking about the deceased, often beginning with the more positive memories before exploring areas where there may have been conflict or ambivalence about the relationship. It may also be important to explore earlier relationships, particularly if it is felt that the bereavement has resulted in some recurrence of traumatic events.

In therapy there are often stages or tasks of grieving that the therapist will help the bereaved to explore. All or some of these may need to be addressed. A fundamental first step is making sure the individual has accepted the reality of the loss. If this is a problem, therapy focuses on the reality of the death and developing a complete awareness of the loss in a sympathetic way. In day-to-day practice, this type of reaction is rare and it is more common to see delayed or inhibited grief. In these cases, the therapist allows or encourages the expression of emotion and provides reassurance that this is safe.

A number of bereaved people may feel unable to face particular situations, or make decisions, without the deceased. This can result in difficulties which may include practical problems as well as social isolation. Help for people having difficulties with this stage of grieving is often focused on encouraging the bereaved to lessen feelings of helplessness through problem-solving and trying out new roles or skills.

The last stage of therapy for complicated bereavement reactions is achieved when the therapist helps the individual reduce their emotional attachment to the deceased, and encourages new relationships and getting on with living. This is very different from forgetting the deceased. It involves saying goodbye to the wish that the deceased be alive or recovered in some way. The deceased is removed from playing such a central role in the bereaved person's life.

REFERENCES

Coyle F (1999). Coping with cot death. *Family Medicine* **32**:19–20.
Black D (1998). The dying child. *British Medical Journal* **316**:1376–8.
Kato PM, Mann T (1999). A synthesis of psychological interventions for the bereaved. *Clinical Psychology Review* **19**:275–95.

Websites

Childcare Bereavement
www.childline.co.uk
Provides factsheets on bereavement.

Bereavement Self-help Resources Guide
www.inforamp.net/~bto/index.html
Resources and links.

Self-help

Child Death Helpline
Freephone: 0800 282 986
A confidential helpline for anyone affected by the death of a child. Provides local contacts.

The Compassionate Friends
53 North Street, Bristol BS3 1EN
Tel: 0117 966 5202 (administration)
     0117 953 9639 (helpline)
Website: www.tcf.org.uk
Support and friendship for bereaved parents and their families by those similarly bereaved.

Cruse Bereavement Care
Cruse House, 126 Sheen Road, Richmond, Surrey TW9 1UR
Tel: 0870 1671671
     020 8332 7227 (helpline: 9.30–5.00 weekdays)
     020 8940 3131 (youthline)
Counselling for anyone who has been bereaved, practical advice and social contacts.

Foundation for the Study of Infant Deaths
14 Halkin Street, London SW1X 7DP
Tel: 020 7235 1721 (cot death helpline)
Website: www.vois.org.uk/fsid
Round-the-clock support for parents or others affected by the sudden, unexplained death of a baby. Leaflets are available on request.

SANDS (Stillbirth and Neonatal Death Society)
28 Portland Place, London W1N 4DE
Tel: 020 7436 7940 (office)
    020 7436 5881 (helpline)
Information and a national support network for parents who have lost a baby through stillbirth or neonatal death.

Sibbs
P O Box 295, York YO2 5YP
Email: info@sibbs.demon.co.uk
A national organization run by bereaved brothers and sisters for bereaved siblings. Provides support and information.

chapter 15

The risky patient

IN THIS CHAPTER

- Risk factors for deliberate self-harm (DSH) and suicide.
- Management of DSH.
- Personal safety.
- Recognizing the warning signs of potential violence.

Risk is currently an important topic within mental health. Much of the research in this area has been done in samples of high risk-patients, e.g. repeated self-harmers or those convicted of a violent offence. Evidence from such samples is not readily applicable in primary care where the prevalence of such behaviours is much lower. This chapter will focus on two areas of risk: the self-harming patient and the violent and aggressive patient.

THE SELF-HARMING PATIENT

Epidemiology

Patients who commit suicide and those who deliberately self-harm are separate, but overlapping, groups. It is impossible to make an accurate estimate of the incidence of DSH because many acts of DSH go unreported. As the figures below show, the GP will be in contact with many more patients who deliberately self-harm than patients who commit suicide.

Table 15.1. Epidemiology: DSH and suicide

- 140 000 hospital attendances per year of DSH
- 1% of patients kill themselves in the year following DSH
- 3–5% of patients kill themselves in the 5–10 years following DSH
- 2 in 3 presentations of DSH <35 years

- 5000 suicides per year England and Wales
- 1 suicide per GP every 5 years
- 2% of all male deaths, 1% of all female deaths

Occupations with the highest risk of suicide are vets, pharmacists, dentists, farmers and doctors.

Recognition
Can the GP recognize those patients who are going to self-harm or, more importantly, those who will go on and kill themselves? Risk factors for DSH and suicide are given below.

RISK FACTORS FOR DSH

- Recent episode of DSH.
- Threatening DSH.
- Psychosocial stressors.
- Psychiatric disorder: 2 in 3 do not have a psychiatric diagnosis.
- Alcohol/drug misuse.

RISK FACTORS FOR SUICIDE

- Current suicidal ideas or plan.
- Delusional ideas or auditory hallucinations about harming self.
- Hopelessness.
- Past history of suicide attempts.
- Psychiatric disorder: depression, psychotic illness, personality disorder.
- Alcohol/drug misuse.
- Demographic factors (male, living alone).
- Painful medical illnesses.
- Recent psychiatric hospital discharge.
- Poor compliance with treatment plans.
- Family history of suicide.

Although about a third of individuals who commit suicide consult their GP in the month before taking killing themselves, the event is so rare that no meaningful predictive factors exist. In secondary care, 50% of patients who kill themselves have been seen in the week before death. Although these statistics suggest that suicide prediction is an uncertain science, it does not follow that suicide prevention is a hopeless task. Identifying and attempting to reduce the risk factors for suicide may save lives. Common sense suggests that protective factors, such as children, friends and supports, may act to counter the risk factors – although hard evidence is lacking.

Management in primary care

Many patients are assessed in the general hospital following an episode of DSH. Local services vary greatly in the assessment and follow up provided. Poor compliance with aftercare is, however, common, and the GP may be left without much support in ongoing management.

Management in primary care of repeated acts of DSH consists of:

- Management of associated disorders if present.
- Ongoing assessment of risk.
- Establishment, if possible, of a therapeutic alliance.

Repeated and frequent DSH can lead to feelings of frustration and exasperation. It is important to recognize these feelings and consider how this may be conveyed to the patient either overtly or covertly.

The following acronym may prove a use *aide-mémoire* in managing the patient who repeatedly self-harms. It refers to a general management style rather than any specific intervention, PADS:

- Predictable.
- Available.
- Dependable.
- Supportive.

The adoption of such a strategy may reduce the amount of time spent dealing with minor emergencies and crises. There can be considerable secondary gain for patients who self-harm, and having a more structured approach to care may diminish this.

When to refer

- Concern about suicide risk – consider both the checklist and your gut feelings.
- A change in the presentation of the patient who repeatedly self-harms.

What to expect from secondary care

Most GPs want access to a rapid psychiatric assessment following an episode of DSH to provide an assessment of risk.

There is no fully convincing evidence for the effectiveness of any intervention following DSH. A systematic review of such interventions identified the following services as of potential value:

- Problem–solving treatment.
- Provision of a card to allow patients to make emergency contact with services.
- Depot flupenthixol for recurrent self-harm.
- Long-term psychological treatment for female patients with a borderline personality disorder.

(Hawton *et al.*, 1999)

CASE STUDY: SALLY

Sally was a 35-year-old woman who had been in contact with the specialist mental health services for 5 years following the breakdown of her marriage. She had been engaged in an acrimonious custody battle with her husband over their three children who were eventually placed in the custody of their father. Sally began a pattern of repeated overdoses and cutting, together with increasing use of alcohol. She had had three relatively brief hospital admissions which were not felt to have been particularly beneficial, in that her self-harming often increased during admission. The self-harming was noted to be worse at times of stress, e.g. following access visits to the children, and during legal disputes with her ex-husband and social crises concerning friends and relations.

Sally was seen on a regular basis (every 2–3 weeks) over about a year by a community psychiatric nurse (CPN) and also by her GP, Dr Jones, with the same frequency. Sally's CPN went on maternity leave and the support that Sally received was reduced. Sally began consulting the GP more frequently expressing hopeless thoughts and asking for more help. Dr Jones rang through to the CMHT, but was told that they had not been able to cover the maternity leave and that Sally was not a priority because she did not have a 'serious mental illness'.

Four months after her CPN went on maternity leave, Sally was admitted to hospital following an overdose of 40 paracetamol. She took her own discharge after 4 days. She was found dead on the train line 2 weeks after the admission.

Lessons from the case study

- Patients who deliberately self-harm can be frustrating individuals to support.
- Regular, 'low-grade' predictable support may well be having a role even when self-harming behaviours continue.
- Repeated self-harm is a predictor of suicide as is alcohol misuse, threatening suicide and living alone.
- No clear protective factors.
- Need to develop working links between primary and secondary care to ensure that the experience of primary care is properly noted when management decisions are made.

THE VIOLENT AND AGGRESSIVE PATIENT

Epidemiology

The media have played an important role in stigmatizing the mentally ill as dangerous and menacing. People leaving mental hospitals are reported as 'released' rather than 'discharged'. The language tends to be pejorative, using terms such as 'psycho', 'crazed' or 'madman'.

Homicides committed by patients suffering from serious mental illness have been cited as caused by the failure of care in the community. In fact, on reviewing the homicide statistics 1957–95, there has been only minor fluctuations in the numbers of people with mental illness committing homicide, 'and a 3% annual decline in the contribution to official statistics' (Taylor and Gunn, 1999).

Those who probably fear aggression and violence the most – the elderly – are the least at risk. Those most at risk from violent offending are young men 17–21 years of age. Half of violent crimes occur near to public houses or in domestic disputes. In a quarter of cases, the victim has been a co-participant in the violent episode.

Although serious mental illness is associated with an increased risk of violence, the overall contribution of mental illness to violent offences is only about 3.5%. A specific group who are at high risk to both themselves and others, are patients with severe mental illness and the co-morbid problems of personality disorder and substance misuse.

Recognition

It is just as difficult to predict violent behaviour as it is to predict suicide. The experienced practitioner will know if a particular patient is normally brusque, assertive, irritable, demanding and aggressive. When dealing with an aggressive patient consider, is this different from usual and how does it make me feel? A sense of heightened concern or fear should be noted and acted upon.

When assessing the risk of violence in any situation in the surgery or on a home visit, consider the dangerousness checklist.

THE DANGEROUSNESS CHECKLIST

When assessing the extent of the risk of violence in a situation you are about to enter you should consider the following questions. The more often you answer 'yes', the greater the risk of violence.

- Is the person I am dealing with facing high levels of stress?
- Is the person likely to be drunk or on drugs?
- Does the person have a history of violence?
- Does the person have a history of criminal convictions?
- Does the person have a history of psychiatric illness?
- Does the person suffer from a medical condition which may result in a loss of self-control?
- Has the person verbally abused me or threatened me with violence in the past?
- Has the person attacked me in the past?
- Does the person perceive me as a threat?
- Does the person have unrealistic expectations of what I can do?
- Does the person perceive me as wilfully unhelpful?
- Have I felt anxious for my safety with this person before?
- Are other people present who will reward the person for violence?

(Breakwell, 1989)

Management in primary care

✓ The patient.
✓ The surgery.
✓ The doctor.
✓ Planning community visits.

Factors in the patient

- Identify and treat alcohol and substance misuse.
- Identify and treat psychotic and manic symptoms.
- Stress management and anger management if available.

Factors in the surgery

- Environment: given that patients will often have to wait before being seen, reception areas should be light and airy. The reception staff should be able to see and observe the whole area. Treatment and consultation rooms should provide privacy and, ideally, have silent panic buttons linked to reception staff. Staff should be aware what to do if the alarm is sounded, – get help, call the police and so on. Arrange furniture in clinical areas so that a staff member is nearer to the door than the patient.
- Information: keep waiting patients informed if there are going to be delays, giving them the reasons for the delays.
- Planned consultations: if you are presented with a potentially difficult situation, make the appointment when you have adequate time and when sufficient staff are available. See the patient with a staff member if necessary.
- Effective communication: if at any time during a consultation you feel any sense of threat or menace this should be recorded in the patient's notes. You should not be embarrassed to tell your colleagues of your experience. Information is of little use unless it is shared. It is also of value to maintain a record in the patient's notes if they have convictions for violent crime.
- Training: as a practice and multi-professional group, do you have a strategy for staff training in the problems of dealing with difficult people?

Factors in the doctor

■ Personal presentation: personal style, delivery and body language are how others perceive us. It is not what you say, but the way that you say it. Although an authority figure, the GP does not have to be authoritarian. When talking to angry people, Shepherd (1994) advises:
  - pay close attention; stand outside their personal space and slightly out of their arms' reach,
  - adopt a quiet, calm, but determined, manner,
  - use calm body language; adopt a relaxed posture with your hands open; maintain an attentive expression,
  - avoid staring eye contact,
  - avoid pointing at, or touching, angry people.
■ Characteristics of potential victims: am I tired, inexperienced, stressed and running late? Has this made me inflexible, confrontational and more demanding than usual?
■ The consultation:
  - be courteous, relaxed and non-aggressive, whatever the patient's behaviour. Greet them by saying 'Good morning', or similar neutral words and 'How can I try and help you'. Aim to set the scene for a normal consultation,
  - identify signs of arousal in the patient: rapid breathing, clenched teeth, flushing, loud talking, restless or repetitive movements and violent gestures, e.g. pointing,
  - if you are feeling uneasy, stop the consultation. You should not be feeling unsafe.
■ Planning community visits:
  - What are the risks?
  - Am I at risk of a possible robbery because I am known to be carrying drugs?
  - Does the patient or their carer or other family member pose a risk to me if I am unable to meet their perceived needs?
  - Is the patient unknown to me?

IN THE COMMUNITY THE RISK IS GREATER IF YOU ANSWER 'YES' TO SEVERAL OF THE FOLLOWING QUESTIONS

- Am I alone without back-up?
- Are colleagues unaware of my whereabouts?
- Am I without any means of raising the alarm if attacked?
- Am I likely to be trapped without an escape route if the person becomes violent?
- Am I aware of how I react in violent situations?
- Am I unaware of the cultural norms which are likely to control this person's exhibition of violence?
- Have I considered what I would do if attacked?

(Breakwell, 1989)

In Shepherd (1994) there is a useful list of do's and don'ts for home visiting (Table 15.2).

When to refer

- Patients with a history of mental illness and an identified risk of violence to others:
  - all patients with a history of serious violence in the context of mental illness should be kept under review by specialist services.
- Refer to social services child care team if there are any concerns about violence to children whether or not mental illness is present.
- Adult victims of violence may develop mental illness which may need specialist help.

Table 15.2. Do's and don'ts for home visiting

Do	Don't
Dress inconspicuously	Advertise your profession with car stickers and similar items which could be an invitation to drug-seekers
Use a sports bag instead or a 'doctor's' bag	Carry unnecessary equipment or drugs
Know your practice patch	Wander about looking lost, or loiter if you are uncertain where you are
Before a visit, familiarize yourself with your patients' notes and family history	Rely on second- or third-hand reports
Ask to go with a colleague such as a community psychiatric nurse	Be ashamed to ask for support
Ask for a police escort if necessary	Rely on a personal alarm. Who would hear it and who would know what it was?
On arrival try to memorize access and exit routes	Leave yourself with a complicated route back to your car
Use stairs instead of the lift	Hesitate to change your route if you think you are being followed

REFERENCES

Breakwell GM (1989). *Facing Physical Violence.* Routledge, London.
Hawton K, Arensman E, Townsend E (1999). *Psychosocial and Pharmacological Treatments for Deliberate Self Harm.* The Cochrane Library.
Shepherd J (1994). *Violence in Health Care.* OUP, Oxford.
Taylor P J, Gunn J (1999). Homicides by people with mental illness. Myth and reality. *British Journal of Psychiatry* **174**:9–14.

FURTHER READING

Department of Health (1999). *Safer Services. National Confidential Enquiry into Suicide and Homicide by People with Mental Illness.* Department of Health, London.
Woods M, Whitehead J, Lamplugh D (1993). *Working Alone Surviving and Thriving.* Pitman, London.

A useful resource is a recent joint publication from the Royal College of Nursing and the NHS Executive: Safer Working in the Community: A guide for NHS managers and staff on reducing the risks from violence. This publication is available from Department of Health, PO Box 410, Wetherby LS23 7LN.

WEBSITES

Stop Violence to NHS Staff
www.nhs.uk/zerotolerance
A resource pack for the prevention and management of violence towards NHS staff.

The Mental Health Act 1983 England & Wales

Proposals to alter the 1983 Mental Halth Act have been published by the UK government. It is likely, however, that GPs will still be called upon to assist in determining whether their patients need a compulsory admission to hospital.

A patient suffering from a mental disorder may be compulsorily admitted under the Act:

- In the interests of his or her own health, *or*
- In the interests of his or her own safety, *or*
- For the protection of other people.

Section 12 approved doctors are experienced psychiatrists, or GPs with recognized expertise in mental health.

GPs may be involved in four sections of the 1983 Act: 2, 3, 4 and 136. An assessment under the Act will usually be done with an approved social worker and an experienced psychiatrist.

SECTION 2: ADMISSION FOR ASSESSMENT OR ASSESSMENT FOLLOWED BY TREATMENT

Section 2 is used for compulsory admission when a patient is not known to the professionals – diagnosis and prognosis are not clear.

Duration
Up to 28 days from admission.

Grounds
(a) Mental disorder which warrants detention in hospital for assessment, and
(b) Admission is necessary in interests of the patient's own health, or safety, or for the protection of others.

Recommendations
Two doctors, one section 12 approved, must examine the patient within 5 days of each other. The patient should then be admitted within 14 days of the last recommendation. One doctor should have previous knowledge of the patient (usually the GP). The doctor making the second recommendation should not work at the same hospital as the first.

Application
Nearest relative or Approved Social Worker (ASW) must have seen the patient within 14 days of the application.

SECTION 3: ADMISSION FOR TREATMENT

Duration
Up to 6 months, renewable after 6 months and then annually.

Grounds
(a) Mental illness, mental impairment, severe mental impairment or psychopathic disorder, and
(b) The mental disorder is of a nature or degree which makes it appropriate for the patient to receive medical treatment in hospital, and

(c) Admission is necessary for the health, or safety, of the patient, or for the protection of others, and

(d) In the case of psychopathic disorder and mental impairment, treatment is likely to alleviate or prevent deterioration in the patient's condition.

Recommendation
As in section 2.

Application
Nearest relative or ASW must have seen the patient within 14 days of the application. If the nearest relative objects, the ASW cannot make the application. If the objection is deemed to be unreasonable, the ASW can make an application to the county court to override the nearest relative.

SECTION 4: EMERGENCY ADMISSION FOR ASSESSMENT

This section allows a simpler procedure than section 2 and provides the power to detain patients in emergencies.

Duration
Up to 72 hours from the admission of the patient with the understanding that a section 2 will be organized from the time of admission.

Grounds
(a) Mental disorder which warrants detention in hospital for assessment, and

(b) Admission is necessary in the interests of the patient's own health or safety or for the protection of others.

Recommendation
One doctor, preferably with previous knowledge of the patient, within 24 hours of seeing the patient.

Application

The nearest relative or an ASW who must have seen the patient within 24 hours.

SECTION 136: MENTALLY DISORDERED PERSON FOUND IN A PUBLIC PLACE

This section of the Act empowers a police constable to arrest a person who 'appears' mentally disordered in a public place and convey them to 'a place of safety'. The place of safety may be a hospital or the custody area of the local police station. The purpose of detention is to allow the patient to be examined by a doctor who can then make appropriate arrangements for the patient's care.

Index